Congestive Heart Failure:
Pathophysiology, Diagnosis and Management

First Edition

Jon D. Blumenfeld, M.D.

Associate Professor of Medicine
Cardiovascular Center
The New York Hospital – Cornell Medical Center
New York, NY

and

John H. Laragh, M.D.

Hilda Altschul Master Professor of Medicine
Chief, Division of Cardiology and
Cardiovascular Center
The New York Hospital – Cornell Medical Center
New York, NY

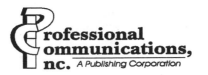

Professional Communications, Inc. *A Publishing Corporation*

Published by:
Professional Communications, Inc.

P.O. Box 10   400 Center Bay Drive
Caddo, OK 74729   West Islip, NY 11795

For orders only, please call:
1-800-337-9838

ISBN: 0-9632400-6-4

Library of Congress Card Number: 93-087072

Printed in the United States of America

Typography by
Iluztrafix—DTP, UnLtd.
P.O. Box 924 • Durant, OK 74702-0924

This text is printed on recycled paper.

Dedication

This work is dedicated to my parents.

Jon D. Blumenfeld, M.D.

To my wife, Jean.

John H. Laragh, M.D.

Acknowledgement

Dr. Blumenfeld is the recipient of a Clinical Associate Physician Grant, Public Health Service Research Grant RR00047 from the General Research Center Branch, Division of Research Facilities and Resources, Bethesda, Maryland. This work is also funded in part by a grant from the William H. Kearns Foundation.

TABBED TABLE OF CONTENTS

FIGURES

TABLES

ix

PART

DEFINITION &
EPIDEMIOLOGY

1 Definition and Epidemiology of Heart Failure

Definition of Congestive Heart Failure

Heart failure is traditionally defined as the pathophysiological state in which the heart is unable to pump blood at a rate commensurate with the body's metabolic requirements. This reduction in myocardial function is most commonly caused by ischemic injury produced by obstructive coronary artery disease, but is also a consequence of primary cardiomyopathy and anatomic lesions of the cardiac valves and pericardium.

During the past decade, compensatory neurohumoral and hemodynamic mechanisms have been identified that maintain cardiac output and peripheral perfusion when cardiac function is impaired (Figure 1.1). Congestive heart failure develops when these adaptive mechanisms are inadequate and progressive deterioration in cardiac performance occurs. The modern treatment of heart failure is directed toward the correction of these pathophysiologic mechanisms.

Epidemiology of Congestive Heart Failure

The National Heart, Lung and Blood Institutes estimates that more than two million Americans are afflicted with heart failure, with 400,000 new cases and 900,000 hospitalizations occurring each year. There are between 200,000 to 400,000 deaths annually attributed to heart failure. Surprisingly, mortality related to heart failure has increased since 1968,

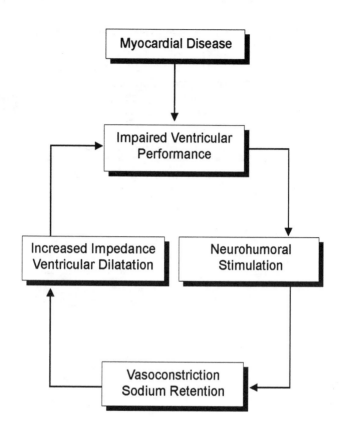

Figure 1.1 — Vicious cycle of heart failure. As cardiac output falls, compensatory responses produce vasoconstriction and elevate systemic vascular resistance, which perpetuates myocardial failure.

Reprinted with permission. Adapted from Cohn J: Drug Treatment of Heart Failure. Stoneham, MA: Yorke Medical Books, 1983;7.

despite the overall decline in deaths related to cardio-vascular disease.

In addition to the cost of human life, heart failure poses a tremendous financial burden on the health care system. In 1990, it was the most common discharge diagnosis in persons over age 65 and accounted for annual expenditures exceeding $4.7 billion. It has been estimated that by the year 2030, the number of persons over 65 will exceed those under 65 and that 2.6 million people will be treated for heart failure.

Therefore, the syndrome of congestive heart failure poses several challenges:

- Who is at risk for developing heart failure?
- Are there risk factors that are remediable?
- How is therapeutic efficacy defined?
- Which forms of therapy are effective?

In this section, the profile of patients at risk for developing heart failure will be outlined.

Risk Profile

The most recent analysis of 34 years of follow-up in the Framingham Study found that advanced age was an important determinant of risk of heart failure (Figure 1.2). The prevalence of heart failure was about 1% for those age 50 to 59 years and rose progressively with age to affect 10% of persons in their 80s. The annual incidence also increased with age, from about 0.2% in persons 45 to 54 years to 5.4% in men 85 to 95 years.

In the Framingham cohort, 37% of men and 33% of women died within two years of their diagnosis in cardiac failure, and after six years, mortality rates increased 82% and 67%, respectively. This represents a death rate from four to eight times higher than that in the general population at the same age. The risk of death increases in parallel with worsening New York Heart Association (NYHA) Functional Class (see Section #7, *The Clinical History*), with 50 to 60% of patients with Class IV dying within one year (Figure

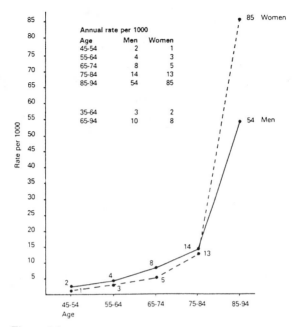

Figure 1.2 — Incidence of cardiac failure by age and sex, 30-year follow-up (Framingham Study).

Reprinted with permission. Kannel WB, Apples A: Epidemiology and risk profile of cardiac failure. Cardiovascular Drugs and Therapy 1988;2:387-395.

1.3). Sudden death occurred in 28% of the men and in 14% of the women in the Framingham cohort, but in other shorter term intervention trials, the incidence has been between 10 and 50%.

With each decade of age, the incidence of heart failure approximately doubles, with women lagging slightly behind men (Table 1.1). This male predominance persists until the ninth decade of age and relates to the presence of coronary heart disease, which in the Framingham cohort, conferred a four-fold increased risk of cardiac failure. Furthermore, the risk of heart failure in men with coronary disease increased from 44 to 50% since 1950. Those with asymptomatic myocar-

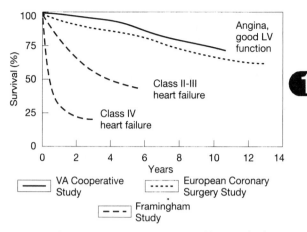

Figure 1.3 — Survival curves for patients with congestive heart failure compared with those for patients with angina and good left ventricular function.

Katz AM: Chairman's introduction. Clinical Cardiology 1993;16(suppl II):II-1–II-4. This figure was reprinted with permission of Clinical Cardiology Publishing Co., Inc.; Box 832; Mawhaw, NJ 07430-0832 USA.

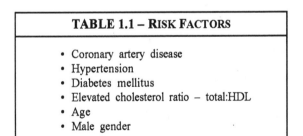

dial infarction were at equivalent risk to those who survived a symptomatic myocardial infarction for one year. In other more recent, controlled therapeutic trials, coronary artery disease accounted for approximately 50 to 75% of cases of heart failure.

In the Framingham Study, hypertension tripled the risk for developing heart failure, with elevated systolic pressure being more predictive of its development. High blood pressure was present in approximately 75% of men and women with heart failure, although a staggering 90% of patients with coronary disease who developed heart failure also had hypertension. The most common diagnostic indicators of increased risk of overt heart failure were:

- ECG evidence of left ventricular hypertrophy
- Sinus tachycardia
- Low vital capacity

"Modifiable" risk factors for heart failure include:

- Hypertension
- Impaired glucose tolerance
- An elevated ratio of total to high density lipoprotein cholesterol
- Obesity

However, despite the 30% reduction in hypertension and 40% decrease in smoking observed in the Framingham cohort during the past three decades, no decrease in heart failure was detected and the risk from coronary disease continued to increase in men. During that period, the risk of heart failure from diabetes also increased significantly.

Causes of Death in Heart Failure

The cause of death is often difficult to determine in patients with heart failure because it can be obscured by the associated chronic symptoms. Deaths are often classified as cardiac or noncardiac (Table 1.2). Those cardiac deaths which are not classified as arrhythmic (because they do not result from ventricular tachycardia or fibrillation), include:

- Myocardial ischemia or infarction
- Progressive pump failure
- Electromechanical dissociation
- Myocardial rupture

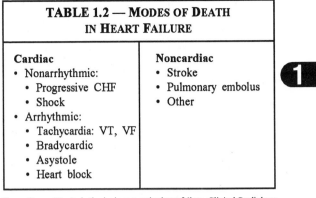

TABLE 1.2 — MODES OF DEATH IN HEART FAILURE

Cardiac	Noncardiac

• Nonarrhythmic:
  • Progressive CHF
  • Shock
• Arrhythmic:
  • Tachycardia: VT, VF
  • Bradycardic
  • Asystole
  • Heart block
	• Stroke
	• Pulmonary embolus
	• Other

From: Greene HL: Arrhythmias in congestive heart failure. Clinical Cardiology 1992;15(suppl I):I-13–I-21. This table was reprinted with permission of Clinical Cardiology Publishing Co., Inc.; Box 832; Mahwah, NJ 07430-0832 USA.

Arrhythmic deaths may result from ischemia or infarction, as well as other etiologies such as electrolyte abnormalities.

Noncardiac deaths may arise from vascular complications such as:
- Stroke
- Pulmonary embolus

Regardless of the etiology of heart failure, mortality rates increase with worsening clinical symptoms and declining left ventricular ejection fraction.

Risk Reduction

(also see Section #11, *Pharmacologic Therapy*)

Although the incidence of heart failure has not been decreased with improved control of risk factors for coronary disease, survival of patients with heart failure has improved modestly with specific treatments. Captopril, an angiotensin converting enzyme (ACE) inhibitor, improves survival and decreases the development of congestive heart failure when treatment is begun shortly after myocardial infarction. In addition, ACE inhibitors improve survival in patients with symptomatic heart failure. Interventions designed to improve salvage of ischemic myocardium and reduce the incidence of lethal ventricular arrhythmias may also decrease the incidence of heart failure and its associated risks, although this latter approach has yet to be proven effective.

REFERENCES

1. Strobeck JE, Sonnenblick EH: Pathophysiology of heart failure: deficiency in cardiac contraction. In: Drug Treatment of Heart Failure, Cohn JN (ed). New York: Yorke Medical Books, 1983;13-34.

2. Packer M: Pathophysiology of heart failure. Lancet 1992; 340:88-92.

3. Ghali JK, Cooper R, Ford E: Trends in hospitalization rates for heart failure in the United States, 1973-1986. Evidence for increasing population prevalence. Arch Intern Med 1990;150(4):769-773.

4. Kannel WB, Belanger AJ: Epidemiology of heart failure. Am Heart J 1991;120:951-957.

5. Kannel WB, Pinsky J: Trends in cardiac failure – incidence and causes over three decades in the Framingham Study. Circulation 1991;17:87A.

6. Yancy CW, Firth BG: Survival in congestive heart failure: have we made a difference? Am J Med 1990;88:1-3N–1-8N.

7. Green HL: Clinical significance and management of arrhythmias in the heart failure patient. Clin Cardiol 1992;15(suppl I):I-13–I-21.

PART 2

PATHOPHYSIOLOGY OF HEART FAILURE

2   Normal Cardiac Physiology

CELLULAR PHYSIOLOGY OF CARDIAC CONTRACTION

Contractile Proteins

Cardiac muscle has a unique cellular architecture that facilitates its role in excitation and contraction. Cardiac muscle cells, referred to as myocytes or fibers, contain myofibrils that span the fiber. These myofibrils are composed of longitudinally repeating sarcomeres which are aligned to give the fiber its striated appearance.

The sarcomere is the major contractile unit of the myocardium, its bands represent interdigitating myofilaments of contractile proteins (Figure 2.1). The anisotropic (A) band is the dark band at the center of the sarcomere which is flanked by two lighter isotropic (I) bands. Myosin, located at the A band, is composed of two fragments:

- Heavy meromyosin
- Light meromyosin

The latter is the site of ATPase activity. There are three isoenzymes of myosin, each with a different heavy chain composition:

- V_1 has high activity and is fast
- V_3 has low activity and is slow
- V_2 is intermediate

The proportions of these isoenzymes will determine the ATPase activity and the contractile characteristics. In the human heart, isoenzymes V_3 and V_2 are most abundant.

11

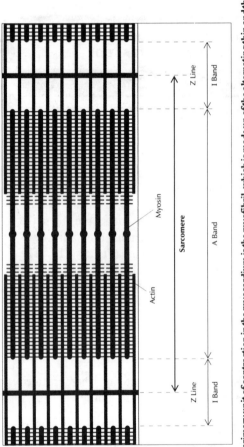

Figure 2.1 — The primary unit of contraction in the myocardium is the myofibril, which is made up of the alternating thin and thick filaments of the sarcomere. Each sarcomere extends from Z line to Z line. Most of the length (the A band) consists of thick-filament myosin. Thin filaments, primarily composed of actin, extend from the Z lines into the A band. The I band includes sarcomere thin filaments not overlapped by thick filaments.

Reproduced with permission. Linderman J: Contractile protein alterations in heart failure. Hospital Practice 1991;26(12):33.

Thin filaments of actin are attached to the Z lines and project into the middle of the sarcomere where they overlap with the thick filaments composed of myosin. Actin filaments, which combine as a double A-helix to form the thin filaments, traverse the region from the Z line through the I band to the A band where they overlap with myosin. Actin is associated with two regulatory proteins, tropomyosin and troponin (Figure 2.2). Tropomyosin is a protein that forms a continuous strand through the thin filament. Troponin, present at intervals along the thin filament, consists of three subunits:

- Troponin C that binds Ca^{+2}
- Troponin I that inhibits actomyosin Mg^{+2}-stimulated ATPase
- Troponin T that attaches troponin to actomyosin

Tropomyosin prevents the myosin heads from binding with actin and thereby inhibits cross-bridge formation during the relaxation phase.

The sarcolemma, or surface membrane, invaginates at the Z line of the sarcomere to form the T system which branches throughout the cell. In close proximity to the T system is the sarcoplasmic reticulum (SR), a membrane enclosed channel that surrounds each myofibril. The sarcolemma is in close proximity to a capillary network and nonmyelinated nerves which release acetylcholine (at the atria and conduction systems) and norepinephrine (at the conduction systems and ventricles). The thickened portion of the sarcolemma, located at the connection of adjacent myocardial cells and termed the intercalated disc, is a low resistance pathway that propagates electrical activity between cells.

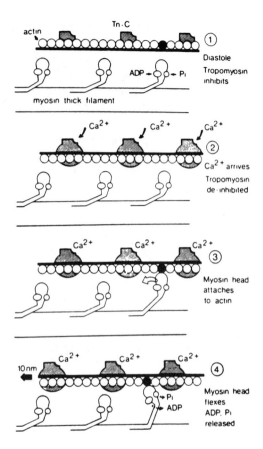

Figure 2.2 — Contractile events in heart muscle. The cross-bridge cycle starts with relaxation in diastole (Step 1) when tropomyosin (Tm), the solid black horizontal line, "blocks" the myosin heads from binding to actin. At the start of systole (Step 2), Ca^{2+} combines with troponin C (Tn-C) so that Tm no longer blocks the actin and so that myosin heads can bind and then "flex," whereupon ADP and inorganic phosphate (P) are released (Step 3). The "rigor state" develops transiently (Step 4). ATP moves in to the same binding site on the

14

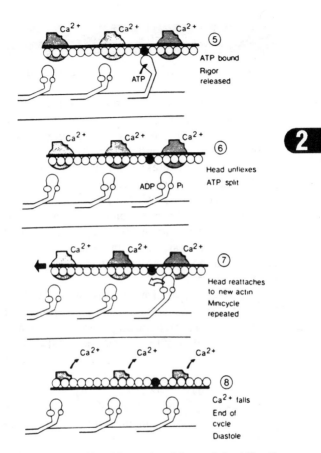

myosin head vacated by ADP, to "release" the myosin head (Step 5). After ATP has been split to ADP and P by the myosin ATPase, the head extends (Step 6) to rebind to another actin 2 to 4 units "downstream" (Step 7). Steps 1 to 7 are repeated until [Ca^{2+}] at the myofiber decreases at the start of diastole (Step 8).

Reprinted with permission. Opie L: The Heart. New York: Grune and Stratton, 1984:101.

Cytoplasmic Calcium

The activity of the contractile proteins is determined by the concentration of cytoplasmic $[Ca^{+2}]$. A 10,000-fold concentration gradient for calcium is maintained across the sarcolemma by several energy-dependent cellular processes. These mechanisms include a Na^+-Ca^{+2} antiporter and an energy dependent calcium pump (ATPase) at both the sarcolemma and SR. During cellular depolarization, when intracellular $[Ca^{+2}]$ increases from 10^{-7} M to 10^{-5} M, calcium binds to troponin C. This causes a conformational change in tropomyosin and, consequently, enhances actomyosin formation. In this way, calcium promotes the interaction between actin and myosin by inactivating an inhibitory effect of troponin.

The force generated during the formation of cross-bridges between actin and myosin is determined, in part, by the degree of shortening caused by the relative changes in position of these filaments and also by the amount of calcium bound to troponin C. Relaxation occurs when calcium dissociates from troponin and is resequestered by the SR through an energy dependent calcium ATPase. Thus, intracellular calcium homeostasis is essential for maintaining the contractile state of the heart.

Adrenergic Activity

The medullary cardiovascular centers regulate:
- Cardiac contractility and rate
- Arterial pressure
- Distribution of blood flow

Tonic activity in these excitatory centers is inhibited by impulses from the baroreceptors. Increased nerve impulse traffic in the carotid sinus and aortic nerves, as well as in cardiac vagal afferent fibers, reflexly reduce efferent sympathetic nerve activity and augment vagal discharges. Consequently, heart rate and vasomotor tone in resistance and capacitance vessels are decreased, and contractility of the atria and ventricles is reduced.

Catecholamine secretion, primarily epinephrine, is stimulated by increased activity of preganglionic sympathetic nerves that synapse at the adrenal medulla. Norepinephrine present in the heart is synthesized and stored in sympathetic nerve fibers.

The effects of sympathetic nerve stimulation or of circulating catecholamines are mediated by membrane-bound adrenoceptors. In the non-failing right and left ventricular myocardium, β_1-receptors account for 80% and β_2-receptors 20% of the total β-receptor population. β_1-receptor agonists (eg, dobutamine) have a predominant positive inotropic effect, whereas β_2-receptor agonists (eg, salbutamol) cause tachycardia. Cardiac α-adrenergic receptors are primarily α_1-subtype; when bound to agonists (eg, phenylephrine) they have a positive inotropic effect. Prejunctional α_2-receptors are also probably present. When bound by an agonist (eg, clonidine), they inhibit norepinephrine release and thereby inhibit the effects of sympathetic stimulation on the heart.

When norepinephrine (or other agonist) is released from a sympathetic nerve terminal, it binds to a β-adrenergic receptor on the myocardial cell membrane (Figure 2.3). It then activates a guanosine nucleotide regulatory protein (G-protein) by allowing GTP to occupy a nucleotide binding site on the G-protein and this, in turn, stimulates adenylate cyclase activity and cyclic AMP (cAMP) formation. Phosphorylation of a variety of protein kinases is a central event in the cellular regulation of contraction (see below). The process is switched off when the intrinsic GTPase activity of the G-protein hydrolyses the attached GTP to GDP. In addition to the stimulatory form (G_s)

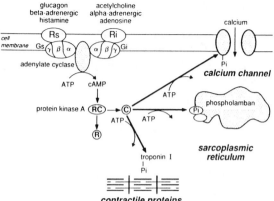

Figure 2.3 — The beta-receptor pathway. Rs, stimulatory receptor; Ri, inhibitory receptor; Gs, stimulatory guanine-nucleotide binding protein; Gi, inhibitory guanine-nucleotide binding protein; R, regulatory subunit of protein kinase A; C, catalytic subunit of protein kinase A.

Reprinted with permission. Lewis BS, Kimchi A: Heart Failure Mechanisms and Management. New York: Springer-Verlag, 1991;17.

described above which stimulates and amplifies signals from the receptors to adenylate cyclase, there is also an inhibitory form (G_i) that attenuates the activation of this enzyme.

Cyclic AMP, acting through the activation of cAMP-protein kinases, is a key second messenger in the regulation of myocardial calcium concentration. Phosphorylation of voltage-dependent (L-type) calcium channels on the sarcolemma increases calcium influx during depolarization and, consequently, increases the force of systolic contraction. β-adrenergic agonists enhance this cardiac Ca^{+2} current via a cAMP-dependent kinase. Conversely, phosphorylation of phospholamban (the regulatory subunit of the sarcoplasmic reticulum calcium pump) increases calcium sequestration and phosphorylation of troponin, decreasing its affinity for calcium and thereby causing relaxation.

18

DETERMINANTS OF CARDIAC PERFORMANCE IN THE INTACT HEART

Preload

The force of cardiac contraction is a function of its preload, defined by its end-diastolic dimensions. This Frank-Starling phenomenon is based on the myocardial length-active tension relation in which the force of contraction is determined by initial muscle length. At the ultrastructural level, this is dependent upon the extent of overlap of actin and myosin filaments within the sarcomere. In the isolated striated muscle preparation, maximum force is generated with a sarcomere length between 2.0 to 2.27 μ. Outside this optimal range, formation of cross bridges is impaired and muscle kinetics are compromised.

In the normal intact heart, ventricular end-diastolic wall stress is analogous to the preload of isolated muscle (Figure 2.4). The relationship between end-diastolic pressure and stroke volume is reflected in the response of the ventricle to changes in ventricular filling (preload) and aortic pressure (afterload). In the intact organism, preload is primarily determined by blood volume and venous return. In addition, atrial contraction increases end-diastolic pressure, thereby augmenting preload and, consequently, raising stroke volume. Improperly timed atrial contraction, such as that which occurs during atrial fibrillation or atrio-ventricular dissociation, decreases preload and compromises ventricular performance.

Afterload

Afterload is defined as the tension or stress (force per unit of cross-sectional area) acting on the ventricular wall after onset of shortening. Several factors determine the afterload, including ventricular volume and

19

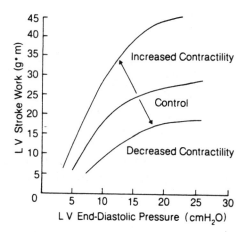

Figure 2.4 — Diagrammatic representation of ventricular function curves expressed as the relation between left ventricular end-diastolic pressure and stroke work. Note that increasing or decreasing underlying myocardial contractility shifts the entire curve as well as changes its shape. It should be noted that the afterload, which can also change the shape and position of these curves, was kept constant during the experimental determination of these curves.

Reprinted with permission. Cohn J: Drug Treatment of Heart Failure. Stoneham, MA: Yorke Medical Books, 1983;14.

pressure, wall thickness and peripheral vascular resistance. The relationship between these variables are expressed in the LaPlace relationship:

$$\alpha = (P \times a) / 2h$$

where:

α	=	circumferential wall stress
P	=	intraventricular pressure
a	=	radius at endocardial surface
h	=	ventricular wall thickness

According to this relationship, wall stress is directly augmented by factors that increase ventricular pressure and volume, and is attenuated when the ventricular wall hypertrophies.

As afterload increases, there is a reduction in stroke volume and velocity of wall shortening. In normal man, during a modest rise in arterial pressure (ie, afterload), stroke volume is maintained by concurrent increases in end-diastolic pressure and volume (ie, preload). If the compensatory increase in preload is attenuated, such as during relative hypovolemia, then an increase in afterload will reduce stroke volume.

Contractility

Contractility, or inotropic state, is a determinant of cardiac performance that is independent from preload and afterload. In a setting where loading conditions are constant, a positive inotropic stimulus increases the velocity and extent of wall shortening and increases stroke volume. Acute administration of negative inotropic agents has the opposite effects. Cardiac contractility can be estimated in the cardiac catheterization laboratory during post-extrasystolic potentiation, the enhanced contraction following an extrasystole. This method provides prognostic information in the setting of regional wall abnormalities that result from ischemic heart disease.

Heart Rate

Heart rate is another determinant of cardiac performance. In normal man, cardiac output is maintained when the heart rate is varied artificially between 60 and 180 beats/minute because of increased contractility. This occurs despite the decrease in the time available for diastolic filling.

REFERENCES

1. Yancy SW, Firth BG: Congestive heart failure. Dis Mon 1988;34:467-536.

2. Braunwald E, Sonnenblick EH, Ross JR: Mechanisms of cardiac contraction and relaxation. In: Heart Disease: A Textbook of Cardiovascular Medicine. Braunwald E (ed). Philadelphia: WB Saunders, 1988;383-425.

3. Morgan JP: Abnormal intracellular modulation of calcium as a major cause of cardiac contractile dysfunction. N Engl J Med 1991;325:625-632.

4. Rosendorff C: Autonomic receptor function in congestive heart failure. In: Heart Failure: Mechanisms and Management. Lewis BS (ed). Berlin: Springer-Verlag, 1991;3-14.

5. Balke CW, et al: Biophysics and physiology of cardiac calcium channels. Circulation 1993;87(suppl VII):VII-49–VII-53.

6. Pereauilt CL, Williams CP, Morgan JP: Cytoplasmic calcium modulation and systolic versus diastolic dysfunction in myocardial hypertrophy and failure. Circulation 1993;87(suppl VII);VII-31–VII-37.

7. Strobeck JE, Sonnenblick EH: Pathophysiology of heart failure: deficiency in cardiac contraction. In: Drug Treatment of Heart Failure. Cohn JN (ed). New York: Yorke Medical Books, 1983;13-34.

8. Grossman W: Cardiac hypertrophy: useful adaptation or pathologic process. Am J Med 1980;69:576-584.

9. Grossman W: Diastolic dysfunction in congestive heart failure. New Engl J Med 1991;325:1557-1563.

10. Anversa P, et al: Cardiac anatomy and ventricular loading after myocardial infarction. Circulation 1993;87(suppl VII);VII-22–VII-27.

11. Pfeffer MA, Braunwald E: Ventricular remodeling after myocardial infarction: experimental observations and clinical implications. Circulation 1990;81:1161-1172.

12. Cohn JN, et al: Plasma norepinephrine as a guide to prognosis in patients with congestive heart failure. N Engl J Med 1984;311:819-823.

13. Ingwall JS: Is cardiac failure a consequence of decreased energy reserve? Circulation 1993;87(suppl VII); VII-58–VII-62.

14. Ferguson DW: Sympathetic mechanisms in heart failure: pathophysiological and pharmacological implications. Circulation 1993;87(suppl VII); VII-68–VII-75.

15. Katz AM: Energetics and the failing heart. Hosp Practice 1991;26:78-90.

16. Bristow MR: Pathophysiologic and pharmacologic rationales for clinical management of chronic heart failure with beta-blocking agents. Am J Cardiol 1993;71:12C-22C.

2

3 Adaptation to Impaired Cardiac Function

The cardiovascular system adapts to the loss of functioning myocardial cells by activating mechanisms that enhance the contractile force of the heart and maintain tissue perfusion. However, long-term activation of these compensatory mechanisms disrupts the normal hemodynamic and neurohumoral balance, resulting in the progressive deterioration of cardiac function.

Compensatory Responses by the Intact Heart

The failing heart depends upon three compensatory mechanisms to maintain its normal function as a pump:

- Increased preload to sustain stroke volume via the Frank-Starling phenomenon
- Myocardial hypertrophy, which increases the mass of contractile tissue and decreases wall stress
- Neurohumoral activation, including increased catecholamine levels to enhance contractility and stimulation of the renin-angiotensin-aldosterone system to increase preload and maintain systemic perfusion pressure (Table 3.1; Figure 3.1)

As with all biological strategies for compensation, these mechanisms have a limited potential and ultimately fail, leading to the syndrome of heart failure.

TABLE 3.1 — COMPENSATION FOR MYOCARDIAL FAILURE

Compensation	Mechanism	Limit
↑ Volume	Length-Tension Curve	Structure of Sarcomere
	Sarcomere	"Fibril Slippage" LaPlace Relation[a]
↑ Hypertrophy	↑ Muscle Mass	↑ Total Force but ↓ force/unit mass
↑ Neurohumoral Activity	↑ Norepinephrine ↑ Renin System ↑ ADH	Volume Overload ↑ Preload, After-load
[a]T = P × R/2h; see text for discussion		

Reprinted with permission. Cohn J: Drug Treatment of Heart Failure. Stoneham, MA: Yorke Medical Books, 1983;22.

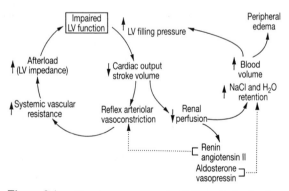

Figure 3.1 — Consequences of impaired left ventricular function.

Parmely WW: Pathophysiology of congestive heart failure. Clinical Cardiology 1992;15(suppl I):I-22–I-27. This figure was reprinted with permission of Clinical Cardiology Publishing Co., Inc.; Box 832; Mahwah, NJ 07430-0832 USA.

Ventricular hypertrophy is an adaptation that preserves cardiac output. The ventricle responds to increased stress, either from volume or pressure overload by initially increasing sarcomere length. However, an excess load results in depressed myocardial contractility. This is manifested *in vitro* by impairment of intrinsic properties of cardiac muscle. Initially, this is due to decreased rate of isometric force development and, as the contractility declines further, by decreased maximum isometric force. In the intact heart, resting cardiac output and stroke volume can be normal, but the ejection fraction is reduced. As contractility decreases further, ventricular volume and/or pressures increase and cardiac output is compromised. At this point, congestive heart failure is clinically apparent.

Characteristic patterns of compensatory ventricular hypertrophy have been described that reflect the type of load applied (Figure 3.2). Cardiac hemodynamics have been compared in patients with chronically pressure-overloaded ventricles with those having volume-overloaded ventricles and equally well compensated systolic function. Left ventricular systolic pressure is significantly elevated in pressure-overloaded but not volume-overloaded patients, whereas left ventricular diastolic pressure is increased in both conditions. However, left ventricular mass is increased in both groups and is more pronounced in the pressure-overloaded patients. Using the law of LaPlace, Grossman demonstrated that in volume-overloaded ventricles, the increased wall thickness (h) was sufficient to counterbalance the increased radius (R), so that the mass to volume ratio (h/R) remained normal for these subjects. In contrast, h/R was markedly elevated in pressure-loaded hypertrophy. Thus, in this concentric hypertrophy typically associated with pressure overload, the increased systolic pressure is offset by increased wall thickness so that wall stress remains

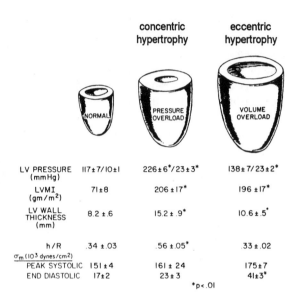

		concentric hypertrophy	eccentric hypertrophy
LV PRESSURE (mmHg)	117±7/10±1	226±6*/23±3*	138±7/23±2*
LVMI (gm/m²)	71±8	206±17*	196±17*
LV WALL THICKNESS (mm)	8.2±.6	15.2±.9*	10.6±.5*
h/R	.34±.03	.56±.05*	.33±.02
σ_m (10³ dynes/cm²) PEAK SYSTOLIC	151±4	161±24	175±7
END DIASTOLIC	17±2	23±3	41±3*

*p<.01

Figure 3.2 — Mean values for left ventricular (LV) pressure, mass index (LVMI), left ventricular wall thickness, the ratio of wall thickness to radius (h/R), and peak systolic and end-diastolic meridional wall stress in patients with normal (6 subjects), pressure-overloaded (6 subjects), and volume-overloaded (18 subjects) ventricles. Although mass is increased similarly in both pressure- and volume-overloaded groups, the increase is accomplished primarily by wall thickening in the pressure-overloaded group. The h/R ratio is normal in volume-overflow hypertrophy, indicating a "magnification" type of growth. In pressure overload, concentric hypertrophy is quantified by the increase in h/R. Patients were compensated with respect to heart failure, and peak systolic tension (σ_m) was not statistically different from normal. However, end-diastolic stress was consistently elevated in the volume-overloaded group.

normal. End-diastolic wall stress was also normal in the pressure-overloaded ventricle, but was elevated in the volume-overloaded group.

Studies from patients with pressure loaded ventricles (aortic stenosis and hypertension) have dem-

onstrated that wall stress is inversely correlated w
two important determinants of ventricular perfor
ance:
- Ejection fraction
- Circumferential wall shortening

However, there was no correlation of wall stress with
left ventricular mass or ventricular pressure. When
these observations were extended to normal subjects
and patients with congestive cardiomyopathy, similar
relationships were observed. But it was evident that at
any level of wall stress, myocardial fibers in those with
cardiomyopathy shortened with a diminished velocity
and to a lesser extent. From these data, Grossman
suggested that the inverse force-relationship in aortic
stenosis did not represent abnormal contractility, but
rather a mismatch with the applied afterload. Furthermore, inadequate hypertrophy and the subsequent
failure to normalize systolic wall stress would then
result in depressed ejection fraction and congestive
heart failure in patients with a pressure-overloaded
ventricle. Support for this concept is provided by
studies that demonstrate improvement in ventricular
performance in patients with aortic stenosis following
correction of the pressure overload.

The pattern of responses by the volume-overloaded ventricle, observed following creation of an aorto-
caval fistula or clinically in patients with aortic regurgitation, differs from those during pressure overload. In the early stages of volume loading, progressive left ventricular dilatation and left ventricular
hypertrophy occur and the length-active tension relationships of the ventricle remain normal. In this eccentric type of hypertrophy as cardiac dilatation progresses,
stroke volume increases, with each sarcomere functioning at its optimal length, until a volume is reached
beyond which decompensation occurs and symptoms
of congestive heart failure occur.

Diastolic heart failure, defined as increased resistance to left and right ventricular inflow, has also been described in most patients who present with congestive heart failure (Table 3.2). Diastolic heart failure can result from structural (eg, pericarditis, amyloidosis) or physiologic abnormalities (eg, impaired myocardial relaxation). Advanced stages of ventricular hypertrophy are associated with qualitative and quantitative changes in myocardial collagen content resulting in increased passive diastolic stiffness and diastolic dysfunction. Hypertrophied myocardium is also more susceptible to ischemia-induced impairment of diastolic function, manifested by angina and an upward shift in the left ventricular volume-pressure relation, even in the absence of coronary artery obstruction. The related decrease in the rate of early diastolic filling of the ventricles leads to an increased dependence on late diastolic filling. Consequently, the contribution by atrial contraction is magnified in the setting of advanced hypertrophy and myocardial ischemia. This accounts for the decompensation of cardiac function that occurs in these patients with the onset atrial fibrillation.

Ventricular Remodeling After Myocardial Infarction

Changes in ventricular architecture after myocardial infarction, referred to as ventricular remodeling, affect myocardial performance and clinical outcome. Following an infarction, pump function is reduced in direct proportion to the amount of myocardium that is lost – involvement of $\geq 40\%$ of the left ventricle leads to acute congestive heart failure or sudden death (Figure 3.3). During the period of resorption of necrotic tissue, before adequate deposition of collagen has occurred, the infarcted region can thin and elon-

TABLE 3.2 — CONDITIONS INVOLVING DIASTOLIC HEART FAILURE

Condition	Mechanism of Diastolic Dysfunction
Mitral or tricuspid stenosis	↑ resistance to atrial emptying
Constrictive pericarditis	↑ resistance to ventricular inflow, with ↓ ventricular diastolic capacity
Restrictive cardiomyopathies amyloidosis hemochromatosis diffuse fibrosis	↑ resistance to ventricular inflow
Ischemic heart disease flash pulmonary edema dyspnea during angina post-infarction remodeling (scarring and hypertrophy)	impaired myocardial relaxation diastolic calcium overload ↑ resistance to ventricular inflow
Hypertrophic heart disease hypertension aortic stenosis hypertrophic cardiomyopathy	impaired myocardial relaxation diastolic calcium overload ↑ resistance to ventricular inflow activation of renin system
Volume overload aortic, mitral regurgitation arteriovenous fistula	↑ diastolic volume relative to ventricular capacity myocardial hypertrophy, fibrosis
Dilated cardiomyopathy	impaired myocardial relaxation diastolic calcium overload myocardial hypertrophy, fibrosis
Obliterative cardiomyopathy endocardial fibroelastosis Loeffler's syndrome	↑ resistance to ventricular inflow

Reprinted with permission from the New England Journal of Medicine 1991;325:1558.

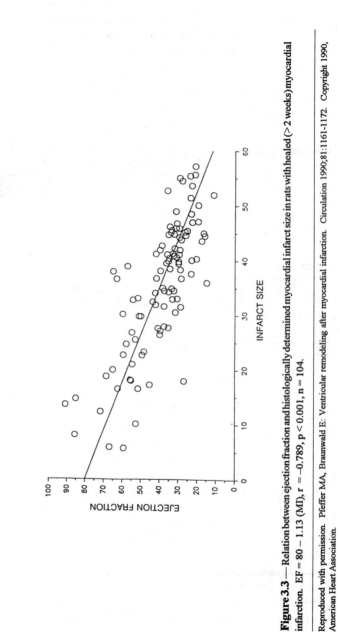

Figure 3.3 — Relation between ejection fraction and histologically determined myocardial infarct size in rats with healed (>2 weeks) myocardial infarction. EF = 80 − 1.13 (MI), r = −0.789, p < 0.001, n = 104.

Reproduced with permission. Pfeffer MA, Braunwald E: Ventricular remodeling after myocardial infarction. Circulation 1990;81:1161-1172. Copyright 1990, American Heart Association.

gate in a process referred to as infarct expansion. Expansion is identified by echocardiography as an akinetic or dyskinetic region, most commonly at the apical-anterior region of the left ventricle.

Concomitant abnormalities of the segment length and contractile pattern of the uninfarcted zone, remote from the coronary occlusion, have also been reported. There appears to be a heterogenous response by myocardial cells depending upon their proximity to the area of scarring – hypertrophic growth in the area adjacent to scarred tissue was reported to exceed that of cells in the portion remote from the infarct. The mechanism for this gradient in the hypertrophic response of the surviving myocardium is not established.

Infarct expansion can occur within a few hours after infarction. Two structural mechanisms have been associated with ventricular dilatation after infarction. One involves the structural rearrangement with side-to-side slippage of cells within the viable and non-viable ventricle. This appears to be an adaptive response to increased diastolic pressure and may be a major influence for mural thinning and ventricular dilatation. In the other pattern of chamber remodeling, increases in myocyte length and fiber elongation have been reported. It is apparent that the changes in chamber volume exceed that which can be attributed to myocyte hypertrophy. As the length of the myocyte exceeds their lateral expansion, a decreased mass:volume ratio characteristic of decompensated eccentric hypertrophy occurs which signals the transition to myocardial dysfunction and failure.

There is abundant evidence in experimental animal models and in survivors of myocardial infarctions that left ventricular volume is a function of both the extent of histological damage and the time after infarction. Progressive enlargement of the infarcted ventricle occurred without increased filling pressure, reflecting a shift in the pressure-volume axis.

Ejection fraction, a measure of global contractile performance, decreases proportionately with the extent of histological damage. Acute compensatory mechanisms, such as the Frank-Starling mechanisms and adrenergic receptor medicated chronotropic and inotropic activity, are inadequate to maintain stroke volume when the non-contractile region involves more than 20% of the left ventricular circumference. Chronic chamber dilatation may restore stroke volume despite reduced ejection fraction, but this is achieved at the expense of increases in wall stress and therefore leads to further ventricular enlargement.

Cardiac enlargement, when observed radiographically in survivors of a myocardial infarction, is associated with a poor prognosis. In this setting, cardiomegaly on chest x-ray has been associated with a three-fold increase in mortality and more than a 15-fold increase in symptoms of severe angina and/or heart failure. Furthermore, survival after infarction is inversely correlated with left ventricular end-systolic and end-diastolic volumes. Left ventricular volume has been reported to be a more powerful predictor of reduced survival than the extent of coronary artery disease. Therapy which decreases afterload and end-diastolic pressure (preload), specifically with ACE inhibitors, has been shown to limit the extent of ventricular remodeling and improve survival following myocardial infarction (see Section #11, *Pharmacologic Treatment*).

Autonomic Function

Heart failure is characterized by increased activity of the autonomic nervous system. The arterial norepinephrine concentration, an index of the activity of this system, is two to three times higher than in normal subjects (Figure 3.4). This is a consequence of increased release and reduced clearance from adrenergic

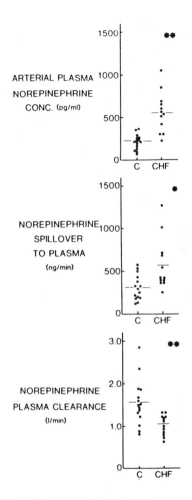

Figure 3.4 — Plasma norepinephrine (NE) concentration and its determinants in control subjects (C) and in patients with congestive heart failure (CHF). The elevated NE level is related to both increased spillover into the plasma and reduced clearance. *p < .02; **p < .002.

Reproduced with permission. Hasking GJ, Esler MD, Jennings GL, et al: Norepinephrine spillover to plasma in patients with congestive heart failure: evidence of increased overall and cardiorenal sympathetic nervous activity. Circulation 1986;73:618. Copyright 1986, American Heart Association.

nerves, leading to "spillover" into the peripheral circulation. This occurs at rest and during submaximal exercise, but not during maximal exertion when normal subjects had higher NE levels, suggesting a relative attenuation of adrenergic drive under maximal stress. However, cardiac stores of norepinephrine are decreased in heart failure, indicating that peripheral sympathetic nerves are its source. Elevated epinephrine levels have also been reported, pointing to increased secretion by the adrenal medulla.

The magnitude of elevation of plasma norepinephrine is directly related to the degree of left ventricular dysfunction as determined by:
- Pulmonary capillary wedge pressure
- Cardiac index
- Left ventricular ejection time

Marked elevations in NE carry an ominous prognosis in heart failure, as the mortality rate increases together with the norepinephrine levels (see below).

Baroreceptor reflex control of cardiac function and the peripheral circulation is impaired in heart failure. Normally, unloading of the baroreceptors, by decreasing blood pressure or lowering blood pressure, increases sympathetic outflow and reduces vagal transmission from medullary centers. This defends blood pressure through positive inotropic and chronotropic effects which increase vasoconstriction and peripheral vascular resistance. These responses are blunted in heart failure. During upright tilt:
- Heart rate does not increase appropriately
- Vasoconstriction is attenuated
- In some patients, vasodilatation of peripheral vascular beds leads to hypotension

Several mechanisms have been postulated to cause the abnormal baroreceptor-mediated responses in heart failure, including:

- Structural and/or biochemical abnormalities of the baroreceptors
- Altered compliance of vascular structures containing the mechanosensory nerve endings
- Abnormality of central nervous system processing of afferent impulses
- Impaired responses to the efferent signal

Recent studies suggest that Na-K ATPase activity is abnormally increased in baroreceptor terminals, thereby hyperpolarizing the baroreceptor and reducing its sensitivity. Digitalis, which has traditionally been considered to exert its beneficial effects in heart failure through its inotropic effects, has recently been shown to normalize afferent baroreceptor function, perhaps via this effect on Na-K ATPase.

The impaired baroreceptor function and excess circulating catecholamine levels found in advanced heart failure are components of generalized neuroendocrine dysfunction that is characteristic of this disorder. Other hormone systems which contribute to this neurohumoral excitation include (see Section #5, *Normal Regulation of Effective Circulating Volume*):

- The renin-angiotensin-aldosterone system
- Antidiuretic hormone
- Atrial natriuretic peptide
- Prostaglandins

REFERENCES

1. Yancy SW, Firth BG: Congestive heart failure. Dis Mon 1988;34:467-536.

2. Braunwald E, Sonnenblick EH, Ross JR: Mechanisms of cardiac contraction and relaxation. In: Heart Disease: A Textbook of Cardiovascular Medicine. Braunwald E (ed). Philadelphia: WB Saunders, 1988;383-425.

3. Morgan JP: Abnormal intracellular modulation of calcium as a major cause of cardiac contractile dysfunction. N Engl J Med 1991;325:625-632.

4. Rosendorff C: Autonomic receptor function in congestive heart failure. In: Heart Failure: Mechanisms and Management. Lewis BS (ed). Berlin: Springer-Verlag, 1991;3-14.

5. Balke CW, et al: Biophysics and physiology of cardiac calcium channels. Circulation 1993;87(suppl VII):VII-49–VII-53.

6. Pereauilt CL, Williams CP, Morgan JP: Cytoplasmic calcium modulation and systolic versus diastolic dysfunction in myocardial hypertrophy and failure. Circulation 1993;87(suppl VII):VII-31–VII-37.

7. Strobeck JE, Sonnenblick EH: Pathophysiology of heart failure: deficiency in cardiac contraction. In: Drug Treatment of Heart Failure. Cohn JN (ed). New York: Yorke Medical Books, 1983;13-34.

8. Grossman W: Cardiac hypertrophy: useful adaptation or pathologic process. Am J Med 1980;69:576-584.

9. Grossman W: Diastolic dysfunction in congestive heart failure. New Engl J Med 1991;325:1557-1563.

10. Anversa P, et al: Cardiac anatomy and ventricular loading after myocardial infarction. Circulation 1993;87(suppl VII):VII-22–VII-27.

11. Pfeffer MA, Braunwald E: Ventricular remodeling after myocardial infarction: experimental observations and clinical implications. Circulation 1990;81:1161-1172.

12. Cohn JN, et al: Plasma norepinephrine as a guide to prognosis in patients with congestive heart failure. N Engl J Med 1984;311:819-823.

13. Ingwall JS: Is cardiac failure a consequence of decreased energy reserve? Circulation 1993;87(suppl VII):VII-58–VII-62.

14. Ferguson DW: Sympathetic mechanisms in heart failure: pathophysiological and pharmacological implications. Circulation 1993;87(suppl VII):VII-68–VII-75.

15. Katz AM: Energetics and the failing heart. Hosp Practice 1991;26:78-90.

16. Bristow MR: Pathophysiologic and pharmacologic rationales for clinical management of chronic heart failure with beta-blocking agents. Am J Cardiol 1993;71:12C-22C.

4   Cellular Pathophysiology in CHF

Considerable attention has been focused on the cellular mechanisms responsible for the abnormalities of excitation-contraction coupling associated with heart failure. Areas of particular interest include:

- Derangements in the regulation of calcium homeostasis
- The imbalance between myocardial energy production and utilization
- Alterations in structure and function of contractile proteins

Abnormal Calcium Homeostasis

Human heart failure has been associated with abnormal handling of intracellular calcium (Figure 4.1). Calcium transients, isometric contractions and action potentials have been measured in patients with normal hearts and in those with hypertrophic and dilated cardiomyopathies. Normally, the myocardial cell calcium signal associated with systole consists of a single peak which declines before peak tension occurs. In patients with cardiomyopathy, the calcium transients were abnormally prolonged, with a delay in the decline of the cytosolic ionized calcium concentration in diastole. In addition, two distinct components of the calcium signal were observed. When extracellular calcium concentrations were increased, the duration of contraction was prolonged and end-diastolic levels of tension occurred in myopathic, but not in normal heart. These findings suggest that myopathic

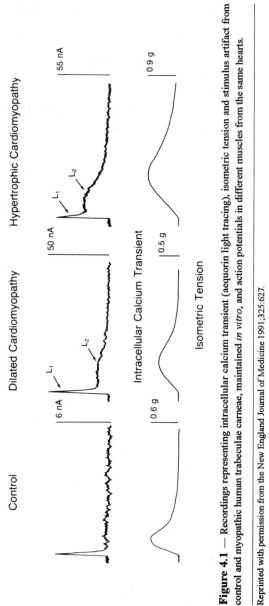

Figure 4.1 — Recordings representing intracellular calcium transient (aequorin light tracing), isometric tension and stimulus artifact from control and myopathic human trabeculae carneae, maintained *in vitro*, and action potentials in different muscles from the same hearts.

Reprinted with permission from the New England Journal of Medicine 1991;325:627.

hearts have an impaired ability to maintain calcium homeostasis in the presence of normal or increased transsarcolemmal gradients. One factor that may contribute to the abnormal calcium handling in patients with cardiomyopathy is the decreased calcium pump activity at the sarcoplasmic reticulum, which is responsible for the sequestration of intracellular calcium during diastole.

Abnormal Responsiveness of Myofilaments to Calcium

In general, the degree of activation of the myofilaments is directly related to the binding of calcium to troponin C. However, this relationship can be modified in a variety of pathophysiologic and pharmacologic states. The responsiveness of the myofilaments to calcium is:

- Decreased during ischemia and acidosis
- Increased during alkalosis

However, increases in intracellular calcium do not necessarily result in increased cardiac performance (Figure 4.2). For example, during ischemia, increases in ionized calcium are associated with impaired systolic and diastolic function. Therefore, it is apparent that other mechanisms contribute to the regulation of cardiac contractility.

In the normal ventricle, ATP concentration is maintained at a relatively constant level. This is a reflection of the numerous pathways involved in ATP biosynthesis including:

- Phosphoryl transfer from phosphocreatine (PCr) catalyzed by creatine kinase
- Substrate level phosphorylation of ADP by oxidative phosphorylation
- Glycolysis

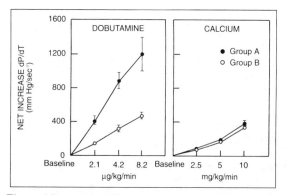

Figure 4.2 — Peak dP/dT responses to dobutamine and calcium in control subjects with left ventricular ejection fraction > 40% (Group A) and patients with idiopathic dilated cardiomyopathy, and left ventricular ejection fraction < 20% and a 50% reduction in β-adrenergic receptor density (group B).

Reprinted with permission from the American Journal of Cardiology 1993;71:26C.

As a consequence of these and other redundant biosynthetic pathways, myocardial ATP content remains constant whereas its synthesis can be adjusted to match the metabolic demand.

Several physiologic and histologic observations have led to the hypothesis that heart failure is associated with an inadequate myocardial energy supply. Phosphocreatine and ATP levels are reportedly decreased in the overloaded ventricle in heart failure. Furthermore, in response to aortic constriction, the fraction of myocyte volume occupied by mitochondria decreases so that there is an increase in the number of myofibrils to be supplied for each mitochondria.

These observations relate to excitation-contraction coupling because contraction and relaxation both require energy expenditure. As described earlier in this chapter, during systole the formation of crossbridges between actin and myosin require energy from ATP hydrolysis. During diastole, ATP is required to bind to myosin to promote dissociation of those cross-bridges. ATP also provides the substrate for the calcium pump (Ca-ATPase) of the sarcoplasmic reticulum as well as other membrane pumps (ie, Na-K-ATPase) and indirectly regulates secondary active transport processes (ie, Na-Ca and Na-H antiporters). Thus, ATP has a dual role in the cellular control of the cardiac cycle:

- As a regulatory or allosteric compound
- As a substrate for a variety of energy dependent processes

Calcium sequestration during diastole in the normal heart is an energy dependent process. Therefore it occurs at a slower rate than calcium delivery, which proceeds down an electrochemical gradient from the extracellular space and sarcoplasmic reticulum to the cytoplasm. An energy deficit, caused by decreased levels of PCr and/or ATP, together with decreased numbers of Ca pumps in the sarcoplasmic reticulum, may explain the abnormalities in intracellular calcium metabolism and contractile kinetics observed in the failing heart. Furthermore, the related abnormalities in ion transport could adversely affect resting membrane potential and thereby increase the potential for arrhythmia.

Impaired Regulation of β-adrenergic Receptors

Heart failure is associated with significant alterations in the myocardial adrenergic receptor-G protein-adenylate cyclase (RGC complex). Changes in adrenoceptor number and affinity have been demonstrated. Down-regulation of myocardial β_1-adrenoceptors has been described in heart failure of several different etiologies, with the degree of down-regulation being directly related to the severity of ventricular dysfunction. Furthermore, this decrease in β_1-adrenoceptors is associated with an impaired contractile response to β-adrenergic agonists. In addition, an increase in G_i has been reported, which may contribute to the decreased cAMP concentration and abnormal regulation of intracellular calcium in the failing heart.

REFERENCES

1. Yancy SW, Firth BG: Congestive heart failure. Dis Mon 1988;34:467-536.

2. Braunwald E, Sonnenblick EH, Ross JR: Mechanisms of cardiac contraction and relaxation. In: Heart Disease: A Textbook of Cardiovascular Medicine. Braunwald E (ed). Philadelphia: WB Saunders, 1988;383-425.

3. Morgan JP: Abnormal intracellular modulation of calcium as a major cause of cardiac contractile dysfunction. N Engl J Med 1991;325:625-632.

4. Rosendorff C: Autonomic receptor function in congestive heart failure. In: Heart Failure: Mechanisms and Management. Lewis BS (ed). Berlin: Springer-Verlag, 1991;3-14.

5. Balke CW, et al: Biophysics and physiology of cardiac calcium channels. Circulation 1993;87(suppl VII):VII-49–VII-53.

6. Pereauilt CL, Williams CP, Morgan JP: Cytoplasmic calcium modulation and systolic versus diastolic dysfunction in myocardial hypertrophy and failure. Circulation 1993;87(suppl VII):VII-31–VII-37.

7. Strobeck JE, Sonnenblick EH: Pathophysiology of heart failure: deficiency in cardiac contraction. In: Drug Treatment of Heart Failure. Cohn JN (ed). New York: Yorke Medical Books, 1983;13-34.

8. Grossman W: Cardiac hypertrophy: useful adaptation or pathologic process. Am J Med 1980;69:576-584.

9. Grossman W: Diastolic dysfunction in congestive heart failure. New Engl J Med 1991;325:1557-1563.

10. Anversa P, et al: Cardiac anatomy and ventricular loading after myocardial infarction. Circulation 1993;87(suppl VII):VII-22–VII-27.

11. Pfeffer MA, Braunwald E: Ventricular remodeling after myocardial infarction: experimental observations and clinical implications. Circulation 1990;81:1161-1172.

12. Cohn JN, et al: Plasma norepinephrine as a guide to prognosis in patients with congestive heart failure. N Engl J Med 1984;311:819-823.

13. Ingwall JS: Is cardiac failure a consequence of decreased energy reserve? Circulation 1993;87(suppl VII):VII-58–VII-62.

14. Ferguson DW: Sympathetic mechanisms in heart failure: pathophysiological and pharmacological implications. Circulation 1993;87(suppl VII):VII-68–VII-75.

15. Katz AM: Energetics and the failing heart. Hosp Practice 1991;26:78-90.

16. Bristow MR: Pathophysiologic and pharmacologic rationales for clinical management of chronic heart failure with beta-blocking agents. Am J Cardiol 1993;71:12C-22C.

4

PART 3

SODIUM AND VOLUME HOMEOSTASIS

5 Normal Regulation of Effective Circulating Volume

Body volume varies directly with total body sodium because sodium is the primary extracellular solute which acts to hold water within the extracellular space. The kidney regulates the excretion of sodium and water and, therefore, plays a central role in maintaining volume homeostasis through a process that involves the integration of afferent receptors and effector systems. The effective circulating fluid (ECF) volume is a component of blood volume to which the volume-regulatory system responds by modulating renal sodium and water excretion.

Although ECF is not a measurable parameter, it reflects the relation between cardiac output and peripheral arterial vascular resistance. If afferent volume (ie, stretch) receptors located in the arterial tree sense an increase in ECF, then the kidneys should respond by excreting increased amounts of sodium and water. However, the arterial blood volume normally accounts for only 15% of total blood volume. Thus, a decrease in arterial volume (ie, filling pressure), relative to the venous component that is caused by a decreased cardiac output, can lead to an inaccurate perception of body volume and set in motion increased reabsorption of sodium and water by the kidney. This then promotes:

- Further increases in venous and intracapillary hydrostatic pressures
- Accumulation of interstitial fluid
- Further embarrassment of the compromised heart, and
- Ultimately, symptomatic congestive heart failure

This chapter will review the processes that regulate volume regulation and illustrate their role in the pathophysiology of heart failure.

Afferent Mechanisms of Volume Regulation — Volume Receptors

Volume receptors are located in:
- The cardiopulmonary circulation
- Carotid sinuses and aortic arch
- The kidney afferent arterioles (baroreceptors) and distal tubules (flow receptors)

These receptors respond to volume-related changes in mechanical stretch or transmural pressure. For example, the intrathoracic low-pressure sensors (ie, atrial, juxtapulmonary capillary [J receptors]) respond to decreased central venous pressure during volume depletion by activating the sympathetic nervous system and a variety of hormonal effector systems that stimulate renal sodium and water reabsorption. Extrathoracic high-pressure arterial baroreceptors located at the juxtaglomerular apparatus perceive changes in renal perfusion pressure and respond by regulating secretion of renin and, thus levels of the sodium retaining hormones:
- Angiotensin II
- Aldosterone

In addition, the kidney regulates sodium and volume reabsorption through changes in glomerular capillary and interstitial pressures that occur in concert with changes in ECF (see below).

Efferent Mechanisms of Volume Regulation — Role of the Kidney

The function of the kidney is to maintain an environment that is optimal for the organism. To achieve this goal, the kidney regulates the excretion of water, electrolytes and waste products through the tightly controlled balance of:

- Filtration
- Reabsorption
- Secretion

These processes are governed, in part, by a variety of hormones, locally operating transmitters and vasoactive substances secreted by the kidney.

In heart failure, the ability of the kidney to regulate these processes appropriately is impaired. This leads to:

- Sodium retention
- Edema
- Further decompensation of cardiac function

As an understanding of kidney function is essential to comprehend the pathophysiology of heart failure, this chapter will review basic aspects of glomerular and tubular function in relation to the maintenance of fluid and electrolyte balance in normal man and in a patient with heart failure.

Regulation of Glomerular Ultrafiltration

Under resting conditions, the blood flow to the kidney is approximately 20% of the cardiac output. When expressed as flow per tissue weight, renal blood flow (RBF) is eight times greater than coronary blood flow. This reflects the low resistance of the renal circulation.

The functional subunit of the kidney is the nephron. Each human kidney is composed of approximately one million nephrons, although there is significant variability in this number among individuals. The nephron consists of vascular and tubular components. The microvascular arrangement is that of two arterioles (afferent and efferent) in series across the glomerular capillary. Blood enters the kidney through serial branches of the renal artery (interlobar, arcuate, interlobular arteries) and enters the glomeruli through the afferent arterioles. Approximately 20% of the plasma reaching the glomeruli is filtered into renal tubules. The plasma which is not filtered exits the glomerulus through the efferent arteriole into the postglomerular capillaries. In nephrons located in the kidney cortex, these capillaries travel in close proximity to the tubules and modulate solute and water reabsorption by the kidney. In juxtamedullary nephrons located deeper in the medulla, the efferent arterioles branch out to form vasa recta which participate in the countercurrent mechanism through which urine is highly concentrated and body water conserved.

The glomerular circulation promotes ultrafiltration of large volumes of fluid due to the excess transcapillary hydraulic pressure relative to oncotic pressure. The rate at which glomerular filtration proceeds is a result of these opposing forces and can be expressed in the following equation:

$$\text{GFR} = K_f \left[\, (P_{gc} - P_{BS}) - (\pi_{gc} - \pi_{BS}) \, \right]$$

$$= K_f \left(\Delta P - \Delta \Pi \right)$$

where:

GFR = glomerular filtration rate

K_f = glomerular ultrafiltration coefficient; related to the total surface area and water permeability of the capillary membrane

P_{gc} = glomerular capillary pressure
P_{BS} = Bowman's space pressure
π_{gc} = glomerular colloid osmotic pressure
π_{BS} = colloid osmotic pressure of the filtrate

Normally, the size and charge characteristics of the glomerular membrane are highly restrictive against the filtration of proteins and so the colloid osmotic pressure of the glomerular filtrate is negligible. Experimental studies have shown that P_{gc} and P_{BS} remain relatively constant along the length of the glomerulus, whereas π_{gc} increases progressively because of the filtration of protein-free fluid into Bowman's space (Figure 5.1). As π_{gc} increases without accompanying changes in P_{gc}, the glomerular transcapillary pressure gradient decreases progressively from approximately 15 mmHg (at the afferent arteriole) towards zero (at the efferent arteriole).

5

The point at which filtration ceases is called filtration pressure equilibrium. During filtration pressure equilibrium, if renal plasma flow (RPF) decreases, there is more time for fluid transfer across the glomerular capillary. As a result, π_{gc} increases rapidly, net filtration pressure is dissipated more proximally along the glomerular capillary, and GFR is decreased. It occurs at low RPF and is important because, in this setting, GFR is flow dependent and changes in proportion to changes in plasma flow.

Since the glomerulus is located between the afferent and efferent arterioles, selective changes in the arteriolar resistances that are caused by vasoactive substances will have a significant impact on glomerular hemodynamics (Figure 5.2). Afferent arteriolar vasoconstriction decreases both GFR and glomerular plasma flow. When the afferent arteriole dilates, more arterial perfusion pressure is transmitted to the glomerulus, and both capillary flow and GFR increase. In contrast, a selective increase in efferent arteriolar

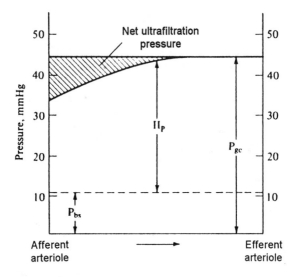

Figure 5.1 — Depiction of the hemodynamic forces along the length of the primate glomerular capillary. The dotted line represents the hydraulic pressure in Bowman's space P_{BS}. The plasma oncotic pressure is added to this so that the middle solid line represents the sum of the forces retarding filtration: $P_{BS} + \pi_p$. The upper solid line represents the glomerular hydrostatis pressure P_{gc}, and the shaded area depicts the net gradient favoring filtration, $P_{gc} - P_{BS} - \pi_p$, which is +13 mmHg at the afferent arteriole. As a result of ultrafiltration of protein-free fluid, π_p increases until the filtration gradient is abolished and filtration ceases. This is in contrast to muscle capillaries where filtration is limited by a decline in capillary hydraulic pressure.

Rose BD: Clinical Physiology of Acid-base and Electrolyte Disorders, 3rd edition, 1989;51. Reprinted with permission from McGraw-Hill, Inc.

resistance reduces glomerular plasma flow but increases glomerular pressure and, thus, GFR increases. This augmentation of GFR by efferent constriction will be limited by the associated decrease in plasma flow and the increase in plasma oncotic pressure.

At the level of the whole kidney, arteriolar resistance accounts for approximately 85% of the total renal vascular resistance. The relation between these pa-

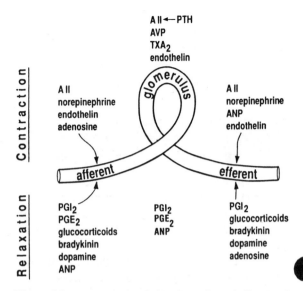

Figure 5.2 — Hormones regulating glomerular and afferent and efferent arteriolar contractility. TXA_2 = Thromboxane A_2; AII = angiotensin II; PTH = parathyroid hormone; AVP = vasopressin; ANP = atrial natriuretic peptide.

Reprinted with permission. Schrier RW, Gottschalk CW: Diseases of the Kidney, 5th edition, Volume I;288. Little, Brown and Company, Copyright 1993.

rameters and RPF can be expressed in the following equation:

$$RPF = \frac{\text{aortic pressure} - \text{renal venous pressure}}{\text{renal vascular resistance}}$$

Accordingly, increases in either afferent or efferent arteriolar tone will increase resistance and decrease RPF. However, the relation between RPF and GFR depends upon whether the predominant change in tone occurs at the afferent or efferent arteriole. GFR and RPF change in parallel during afferent constriction and so no change occurs in the filtration fraction, defined as the ratio GFR:RPF. In contrast, during efferent constriction, reciprocal changes in GFR and RPF occur. This change in the ratio of GFR:RPF signifies that, in general, a change in the filtration fraction accompanies constriction of the efferent but not afferent arteriole.

Role of Peritubular Capillaries in Fluid Reabsorption

Approximately 99% of the 180 liters of glomerular filtrate that is formed each day is reabsorbed by the renal tubules, where it subsequently enters the postglomerular circulation. Reabsorption of fluid by peritubular capillaries is analogous to the process of filtration described above, as it is the net result of an imbalance of hydrostatic and osmotic forces between the interstitial space and capillaries (Figure 5.3). This relationship can be expressed as follows:

$$PR = K_f [(\Pi_c - \Pi_i) - (P_c - P_i)]$$

where:

K_f = reabsorptive coefficient
Π_c = capillary osmotic pressure
Π_i = interstitial fluid osmotic pressure
P_c = capillary fluid hydrostatic pressure
P_i = interstitial fluid hydrostatic pressure

The Π_i and P_i are approximately equal (approximately 6 to 8 mmHg) and therefore tend to cancel each other out. In contrast, as plasma emerges from the efferent arteriole, it has a higher colloid osmotic pressure (35 mmHg) and lower hydrostatic pressure (20 mmHg) than when it entered the glomerulus. Consequently, there is a net reabsorptive force at the initial portion of the peritubular capillary. Fluid is

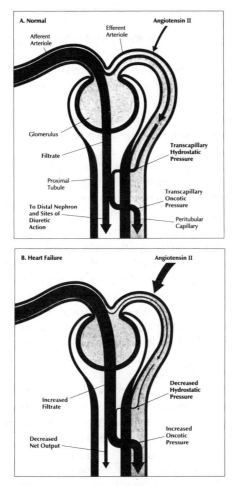

Figure 5.3 — Compared with normal glomerular function (A), that seen in heart failure (B) is marked by an increased filtration fraction, which reduces peritubular hydrostatic pressure, increases the oncotic pressure and thus promotes heightened solute and water reabsorption in the proximal tubule. A key determinant of these changes in the vasoconstrictor angiotensin II, intrarenal and systemic concentrations of which are elevated in congestive heart failure.

Reproduced with permission. Smith TW, Kelly RA: Therapeutic strategies for CHF in the 1990s. Hospital Practice 1991;26(11):73.

reabsorbed along the length of these vessels, with a decrease in II_c accompanied by a small reduction in II_i. Changes in filtration fraction will alter these physical forces and thus influence the rate of peritubular capillary reabsorption. An increase in filtration fraction promotes reabsorption by increasing II and decreasing P; a decrease in filtration fraction attenuates reabsorption. These responses have important implications for edema formation in patients with CHF (see below).

As with glomerular capillary membrane, the peritubular capillary is relatively impermeant to protein. This contrasts with lymphatic capillaries, located primarily in the cortex, which are highly permeable to protein and fluid. Renal lymphatics return protein that has leaked out of the capillaries back to the circulation. Under normal circumstances, the rate of renal lymph flow is only 1% of that of plasma, although it increases in the setting of increased renal venous pressure or other conditions in which interstitial pressure is increased. Efferent arterioles from juxtamedullary nephrons branch to form vasa recta which descend deep into the medulla and are intimately associated with the loops of Henle and collecting ducts. The medullary circulation is characterized by low blood flow and an efficient countercurrent exchange. This system promotes shunting of fluid from descending to ascending limbs while trapping fluid and low molecular weight solutes at a hairpin turn in the inner medulla, after they have been reabsorbed from the tubules.

Renal Tubular Function

(Table 5.1)

■ Proximal Tubule

The proximal tubule reabsorbs approximately 60 to 70% of the glomerular filtrate. Reabsorption by this

TABLE 5.1 — NaCL Reabsorption By Nephron Segments		
Tubule Segment	Percent Filtered NaCl Absorbed	Determinants of Absorption
Proximal tubule	70	Na^+-H^+ exchange Na^+-glucose cotransport angiotensin II norepinephrine peritubular capillary hemodynamics
Loop of Henle	20	Flow dependent AVP
Distal Tubule	5	Flow dependent
Collecting Tubules	4	Aldosterone AVP Atrial natriuretic peptide

Adapted from Bennett CM, Brenner BM: Journal of Clinical Investigation 1968;67:203. Reprinted with permission.

segment is isosmotic and is driven by primarily the Na-K-ATPase pump located at the basolateral membrane (Figure 5.4). This pump maintains a low intracellular sodium concentration and thereby establishes an electrochemical driving force for transepithelial transport of sodium together with other filtered solutes. Sodium entry is passive and occurs electrogenically through luminal channels or can be associated with other solutes by carrier-mediated mechanisms. One example is the Na-H antiporter which is the second most important determinant of proximal tubular sodium and water reabsorption, in addition to its role in bicarbonate reabsorption. Furthermore, angiotensin II directly stimulates Na-H exchange, which accounts

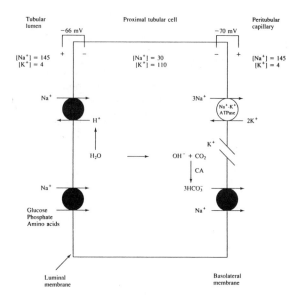

Figure 5.4 — Schematic representation of the chemical and electrical gradients and some of the carrier-mediated mechanisms involved in proximal tubular solute transport. The low cell Na^+ concentration that is maintained by the Na^+-K^+-ATPase pump in the basolateral membrane permits secondary active transport in which passive NA^+ entry into the cell is coupled by specific cotransporters to the uphill reabsorption of glucose, phosphate and amino acids, or to the secretion of H^+. Units are milliequivalents per liter; CA represents carbonic anhydrase.

Rose BD: Clinical Physiology of Acid-base and Electrolyte Disorders, 3rd edition, 1989;91. Reprinted with permission from Mc-Graw-Hill, Inc.

for part of this hormone's action in the regulation of body volume (see below). Fluid and solutes reabsorbed by the proximal tubule enter the intercellular space. Depending upon the peritubular capillary hemodynamics, either reabsorption by these capillaries or leakage back into the tubular lumen may occur.

■ Loop of Henle

The loop of Henle is composed of four segments:
- The descending limb
- The thin ascending limb

- The medullar thick ascending limb (mTAL)
- Cortical thick ascending limb (cTAL)

These segments combine to reabsorb approximately 15 to 20% of the filtered load of sodium.

Fluid entering the loop from the proximal tubule is isotonic to plasma. Unlike the proximal tubule, the thin ascending limb and mTAL are relatively impermeable to water. As sodium is reabsorbed along the mTAL by the Na-K-2Cl cotransporter, the osmolality of the tubule fluid decreases to approximately 50 mosmol/kg as it exits the loop (Figure 5.5). Solute reabsorbed by the loop of Henle of juxtamedullary nephrons accumulates in the medulla thereby increasing the tonicity of the medullary interstitium. This process permits the excretion of a maximally dilute urine during water loading when AVP levels are low, or maximally concentrated urine during dehydration when AVP levels are high (see below).

Approximately 10 to 15% of the filtered load of NaCl exits the loop of Henle and enters this distal nephron. This portion of the nephron includes the distal convoluted tubule, connecting segment, cortical and medullary collecting tubules. It is at this point that the characteristics of the final urine are established, including:

- Magnitude of potassium secretion
- Urinary acidification
- Maximal osmolality

These segments have the capacity to generate large transepithelial concentration gradients but have a limited total reabsorptive capacity, in part because of the lower level of Na- K-ATPase present compared to the proximal nephron segments.

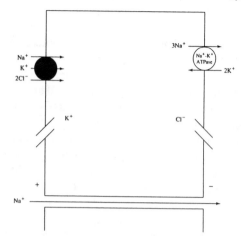

Figure 5.5 —— Schematic model of the major steps involved in NaCl transport in the medullary thick ascending limb of the loop of Henle. Entry into the cell occurs via a passive Na^+-K^+-$2Cl^-$ carrier in the luminal membrane. The energy for this process is indirectly provided by the Na^+-K^+-ATPase pump in the basolateral membrane that maintains a relatively low cell Na^+ concentration. The return of reabsorbed Na^+ and Cl^- to the systemic circulation occurs via the Na^+-K^+-ATPase pump and a Cl^- channel, respectively. Recycling of K^+ across the luminal membrane creates a lumen-positive potential that allows loop Na^+ reabsorption to occur passively via the paracellular route.

Rose BD: Clinical Physiology of Acid-base and Electrolyte Disorders, 3rd edition, 1989;118. Reprinted with permission from McGraw-Hill, Inc.

Cortical Collecting Tubule

This segment is composed of two cell types:
- Principal cells
- Intercalated cells

Principal cells account for approximately 65% of the cells in this segment. They transport sodium and potassium and are important in determining the final urinary concentration of sodium and potassium. The water permeability of these cells is responsive to AVP, allowing them to regulate the osmolality of the final urine.

Reabsorption of sodium occurs through channels at the luminal membrane, down an electrochemical gradient established by Na-K-ATPase (Figure 5.6). Movement of sodium, without an accompanying anion, generates a lumen-negative potential difference and is therefore electrogenic. This creates a driving force for secretion of potassium from the cell into the lumen. As sodium enters the cell, it is exchanged for potassium by Na-K-ATPase and the resulting potassium gradient promotes potassium secretion. When sodium channels are blocked with amiloride, the electrochemical gradient is abolished and potassium secretion ceases. Maneuvers that increase this electrochemical potential, such as high urinary flow (by decreasing luminal potassium concentration) and high serum potassium levels, enhance potassium secretion.

Aldosterone stimulates sodium reabsorption and potassium secretion by the principal cell. This hormone binds to a specific cytoplasmic receptor protein and is then translocated to the nucleus where it interacts with a hormone response element that is present on DNA. Through a subsequent series of steps that are not yet well-defined but which may include the synthesis of aldosterone induced proteins, more sodium and potassium channels open and Na-K-ATPase activity increases.

In contrast to the principal cells, *intercalated cells* in the cortical collecting tubule contain a K-ATPase pump at the luminal membrane. This may contribute to net potassium reabsorption by this segment in the setting of a large total body potassium deficit.

5

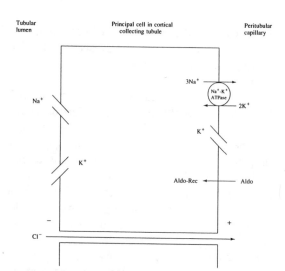

Figure 5.6 — Ion transport in the principal cell in the cortical collecting tubule. Luminal Na⁺ enters the cell through a Na⁺ channel in the luminal membrane. The lumen-negative voltage created by this movement of Na⁺ then promotes either the secretion K⁺ or the reabsorption of Cl⁻ via the paracellular route. These processes are promoted by aldosterone (Aldo), which enters the cell and combines with its cytosolic receptor (Rec). These cells can reabsorb water in the presence of ADH.

Rose BD: Clinical Physiology of Acid-base and Electrolyte Disorders, 3rd edition, 1989;144. Reprinted with permission from McGraw-Hill, Inc.

Medullary Collecting Tubule

This segment of the nephron can be subdivided in outer and inner medullary segments according to their location. The outer medullary collecting duct is composed of cells that function like intercalated cells found in the cortical collecting tubule. These cells have a H-ATPase that can secrete potassium actively and which is responsive to aldosterone. This segment is permeable to water only in the presence of AVP, which promotes equilibration with the hyperosmotic medullary interstitium.

The inner medullary segment contributes primarily toward concentrating urinary maximally. This segment, like the cortical and outer medullary collecting tubules, is permeable to water only in the presence of AVP. However, the cortical and outer medullary segments are impermeable to urea in either the presence or absence of AVP. This differs from the inner medullary collecting duct, in which there is higher basal urea permeability that is increased further by AVP.

Sodium reabsorption occurs in the inner medullary collecting duct through amiloride sensitive sodium channels similar to that described in the principal cells of the cortical collecting duct. In addition, atrial natriuretic peptide decreases sodium reabsorption in this segment by decreasing the number of open sodium channels through a mechanism that is cyclic mediated by cyclic GMP.

Renin-Angiotensin-Aldosterone System

The renin-angiotensin-aldosterone system is a set of interacting and mutually related hormones secreted from the kidney and adrenal cortex, and acting as the major long-term regulator of:
- Sodium balance and extracellular fluid volume
- Potassium balance
- Effective arterial blood pressure

As such, it responds to all influences (external and internal, and particularly dietary salt) that affect any of these three parameters.

The kidneys secrete the enzyme renin in response to a variety of normal and abnormal phenomena that reduce arterial blood pressure, renal perfusion, or sodium chloride load in the distal renal tubule. These include changes in effective blood volume occurring in:

- Sodium depletion
- Shock
- Hemorrhage
- Alimentary fluid loss
- Heart failure

Renin is synthesized by specialized cells, referred to as juxtaglomerular cells, that are located at the afferent arteriole of each nephron (Figure 5.7). The juxtaglomerular cells are in close proximity to the macula densa cells of the ascending limb of Henle and mesangial cells at the hilum of the glomerulus where, together they form the juxtaglomerular apparatus (JGA). Renin secretion is regulated by intrarenal hemodynamic, hormonal and biochemical signals that are integrated at the JGA. These mechanisms that regulate renin secretion include (Figure 5.8):

Macula densa mechanism: It is well established that reduced delivery of sodium chloride to the macula densa stimulates renin secretion and increased loads suppress it. This appears to be a chloride-dependent effect, as other anions with sodium fail to reproduce it. The major determinants of chloride delivery to the macula densa include the filtered load (ie, glomerular filtration rate) and the extent of reabsorption by the proximal tubule and loop segments.

Baroreceptor mechanism: Experimental studies have provided evidence for a baroreceptor in the juxtaglomerular cell that controls renin secretion. Accordingly, stretch of JG cells causes depolarization which increases calcium influx through voltage-sensitive calcium channels. Increases in cytosolic calcium suppress renin secretion, decreases in calcium stimulate it.

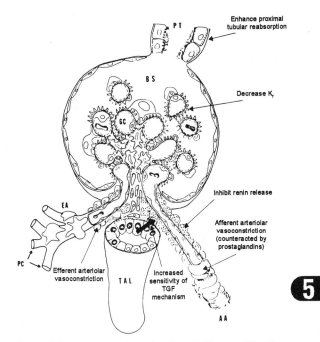

Figure 5.7 — Multiple actions of angiotensin II on renal function. PT = proximal tubule; BS = Bowman's space; GC = glomerular capillaries; EA = efferent arteriole; PC = peritubular capillaries; TAL = thick ascending limb; AA = afferent arteriole.

Reprinted with permission. Schrier RW, Gottschalk CW: Diseases of the Kidney, 5th edition, Volume I;89. Little, Brown and Company, Copyright 1993.

Neural control: Low levels of renal sympathetic nerve activity, which do not alter renal perfusion pressure, stimulate renin secretion. A variety of cardiopulmonary and other reflexes stimulate renin secretion through this efferent pathway. This response is mediated through β_1-adrenoceptors and the related activation of adenylate cyclase and cAMP synthesis. Recent studies suggest that this effect of renal sympathetic nerves may be more powerful than previously considered.

When renin enters the bloodstream it splits off the inactive decapeptide, angiotensin I (AI), from

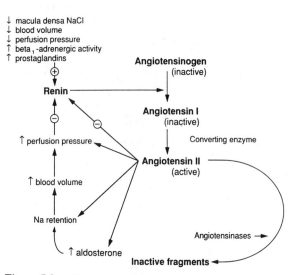

↓ macula densa NaCl
↓ blood volume
↓ perfusion pressure
↑ beta$_1$-adrenergic activity
↑ prostaglandins

Angiotensinogen
(inactive)

Renin

Angiotensin I
(inactive)

Converting enzyme

↑ perfusion pressure

Angiotensin II
(active)

↑ blood volume

Na retention

Angiotensinases →

↑ aldosterone

Inactive fragments ◄

Figure 5.8 — Components of the renin-angiotensin system.

Adapted from Schrier RW, Gottschalk CW: Diseases of the Kidney, 5th edition, Volume I;302. Reprinted with permission from Little, Brown and Company, Copyright 1993.

angiotensinogen (renin substrate). AI is converted to the octapeptide angiotensin II (AII) by angiotensin converting enzyme (ACE), primarily in a single pass through the pulmonary circulation. No role for AI, other than as the precursor to AII, has been identified.

Angiotensin II is the first effector hormone of the renin system. Its actions include (Figure 5.7):

- *Arteriolar vasoconstriction*: AII is bound to a membrane bound receptor, termed the AT$_1$ receptor, located on arteriolar vascular smooth muscle. Subsequent activation of phospholipase C and the related increases in inositol triphosphate and diacylglycerol lead to increased cytosolic calcium. Vasoconstriction occurs in response to this increase in cytosolic calcium.

Other components of AII-mediated vasoconstriction include:
- Synthesis of prostaglandins and leukotrienes
- Inhibition of adenylate cyclase and decreased cAMP formation
- Augmentation by adrenergic activity

- *Renal hemodynamics*: AII decreases renal blood flow and increases filtration fraction, primarily by vasoconstricting the efferent arteriole. However, afferent arteriolar vasoconstriction by AII has been demonstrated. This effect has been shown to amplify the autoregulatory tubuloglomerular feedback mechanism, through which increases in tubular flow lead to afferent arteriolar vasoconstriction.

- *Sodium and water excretion*: In keeping with a basic hemodynamic relationship between arterial pressure and renal sodium excretion, low levels of AII cause sodium retention whereas AII becomes natriuretic with higher dosages or in the presence of arterial hypertension. AII stimulates sodium reabsorption in several ways. First, in response to an increased filtration fraction, peritubular capillary osmotic pressure increases and hydrostatic pressure decreases. Second, binding of low concentrations of AII to AT_1 receptors at the S_1-segment of the proximal tubule stimulates sodium reabsorption via the Na-H antiporter by a process in which adenylate cyclase is inhibited and cAMP levels reduced. In contrast, higher concentrations of AII inhibits sodium reabsorption at this segment. This AII directly stimulates aldosterone biosynthesis and secretion by the zona glomerulosa zone of the adrenal cortex. Fourth, AII promotes thirst and stimulates the nonosmotic release of AVP.

5

cybernetic control mechanism for the maintenance of blood pressure and volume homeostasis has been described, based upon the reciprocal relationship of sodium intake and plasma renin activity. Accordingly, at high levels of sodium intake, intravascular volume, renal perfusion pressure, and macula densa, sodium chloride delivery are normal and renin secretion is not required to maintain blood pressure. In contrast, during sodium depletion, macula densa delivery and renal perfusion pressure are decreased, and efferent renal sympathetic nerve activity is augmented. These multiple effects, dominated by vasoconstriction, combine to raise blood pressure and restore fluid volume to the point where the initial signal for renin release (lowered blood pressure and perfusion in the kidney) is reversed and dampened. The feedback loop has been completed and the renin system's role in maintaining blood pressure and electrolyte homeostasis has been served.

Recently, there has been considerable interest in the possible existence and physiologic operation of local tissue renin systems with novel functions. Prorenin, the biosynthetic precursor of renin, has been identified in ovary, placenta and adrenal tissue where its role as an autacoid has been proposed. However, conversion of prorenin to active renin and secretion of renin occur only by the kidney and plasma renin activity falls to zero after binephrectomy. Therefore, only plasma renin of renal origin has been shown to participate in the cardiovascular responses described above. Thus, plasma renin is the only known activator of the cardiovascular renin system.

Sympathetic Nervous System

Catecholamines play an important role in sodium and volume homeostasis through their direct effects on the kidney and, indirectly, through renin-angiotensin-aldosterone system. Renal sympathetic nerves containing norepinephrine have been identified throughout the:

- Preglomerular renal vasculature
- Glomerulus
- Efferent arteriole

on the:

- Proximal tubule
- Ascending limb of Henle
- Distal tubule

Low frequency stimulation of renal nerves augments renin release through β_1-adrenoceptor activation. At higher frequency stimulation, Na-H antiporter activity and renal sodium reabsorption are amplified by a direct proximal tubular effect of α_1- and α_2-adrenoceptor stimulation. In addition, α_2-adrenoceptor activation promotes sodium and water reabsorption at the proximal tubule in concert with angiotensin II and, in the cortical collecting tubule, enhances AVP-stimulated water absorption. At high levels of renal nerve stimulation, α_1-adrenoceptor mediated vasoconstriction attenuates sodium excretion by decreasing RBF and GFR and, consequently, by increasing renin secretion.

Dopamine is produced by renal nerves and also by the proximal tubule. Low levels of dopamine act through DA_1-receptors to dilate the renal vasculature and promote natriuresis. Higher levels of dopamine cause vasoconstriction and sodium reabsorption by stimulating α- and β-adrenoceptors.

Arginine Vasopressin

Arginine vasopressin (AVP) is released from the posterior pituitary primarily in response to elevated plasma osmolarity. As a result, sodium and water reabsorption is stimulated by the V_2 receptor. This action is mediated by cAMP through an AVP sensitive adenylate cyclase. Nonosmotic stimulation of AVP occurs during marked hypovolemia, where its high levels stimulate the vascular V_1 receptor, leading to vasoconstriction. In contrast to the V_2 receptor, the V_1 receptor acts via the phosphoinositide pathway.

REFERENCES

1. Rose BD: Regulation of the effective circulating volume. In: Clinical Physiology of Acid-base and Electrolyte Disorders, 3rd edition. Rose BD (ed). New York: McGraw-Hill, 1989.

2. Schrier RW: Pathogenesis of sodium and water retention in high-output and low-output cardiac failure, nephrotic syndrome, cirrhosis and pregnancy. New Engl J Med 1988;319:1065-1127.

3. Maddox DA, Brenner BM: Glomerular ultrafiltration. In: The Kidney, 4th edition. Brenner BM, Rector FC (eds). Philadelphia: WB Saunders, 1991;chapter 6.

4. Arendshorst WJ, Navar LG: Renal circulation and glomerular hemodynamics. In: Diseases of the Kidney, 5th edition. Schrier RW, Gottschalk CW (eds). Boston: Little, Brown and Company, 1993;chapter 2.

5. Humes HD, Gottlieb MN, Brenner BM: The kidney in congestive heart failure: with emphasis on the role of the renal microcirculation in the pathogenesis of sodium retention. In: Sodium and Water Homeostasis. Brenner BM, Stein JH (eds). New York: Churchill Livingstone, 1978;1:51-72.

6. Laragh JH, Sealey JE: Renin-angiotensin-aldosterone system and the renal regulation of sodium, potassium and blood pressure homeostasis. In: Handbook of Physiology. Windhager EE (ed). New York: Oxford University Press, 1992;11(section 8):chapter 31.

7. Rabkin R, Dahl D: Hormones and the kidney. In: Diseases of the Kidney, 5th edition. Schrier RW, Gottschalk CW (eds). Boston: Little, Brown and Company, 1993;chapter 9.

8.   Bichet DG, Schrier RW: Cardiac failure, liver disease and nephrotic syndrome. In: Diseases of the Kidney, 5th edition. Schrier RW, Gottschalk CW (eds). Boston: Little, Brown and Company, 1993;chapter 90.

9.   Laragh JH: Atrial natriuretic hormone and the renin-aldosterone axis and blood pressure-electrolyte homeostasis. New Engl J Med 1985;313:1330-1340.

10.   Ballermann BJ, et al: Vasoactive peptides and the kidney. In: The Kidney, 4th edition. Brenner BM, Rector FC (eds). Philadelphia: WB Saunders, 1991;chapter 14.

11.   Luscher TF, Noll G: Endothelium-dependent vasomotion in aging, hypertension and heart failure. Circulation 1993;87(suppl VII):VII-97–VII-103.

6   Derangement of Volume Regulation in CHF

Capillary Mechanisms in Edema Formation

Generalized edema is the result of an imbalance between capillary and interstitial hydrostatic and colloid osmotic pressures. In many tissue beds, local hydrostatic pressures tend to exceed opposing colloid osmotic pressures and, therefore, a gradient favoring filtration is present. The microcirculation utilizes several local mechanisms to defend against edema formation. For example, increases in filtration leads to increase in capillary osmotic pressure and tissue hydrostatic pressure. In addition, vasoconstriction of precapillary sphincters attenuates the transmission of arteriolar pressure.

In patients with congestive heart failure, the development of edema is the consequence of an alteration of capillary hemodynamics, renal sodium and water retention. Disturbances in the local control of the microcirculation that lead to edema include:

- Abnormal pre- and postcapillary resistances
- Increased transmission of venous pressure to the capillary
- Inadequate lymphatic drainage
- Altered permeability of the membrane (K_f) to fluid movement

The mechanisms that lead to sodium and water retention in heart failure are discussed in the following sections.

MECHANISMS OF SODIUM AND WATER
RETENTION IN HEART FAILURE

Afferent Mechanisms

Renal sodium and water excretion is regulated in response to changes in effective circulating fluid volume, as perceived by signals from high pressure (ie, arterial) and low pressure (ie, atrial) baroreceptors (see above). In heart failure, high pressure baroreceptors are activated when cardiac output falls (low output failure) or peripheral resistance decreases (high output failure) to the extent that the arterial circulation is no longer perceived as "full." In heart failure, baroreceptor reflexes are often abnormal and, as a consequence, autonomic regulation of peripheral vascular resistance is impaired. However, the relative contributions of low- and high-pressure baroreceptors in the pathophysiology of heart failure are not well established.

Efferent Mechanisms

■ **Neurohumoral Activation**
Neuroendocrine activation in heart failure is defined by:
- Increased sympathetic nerve activity and plasma catecholamines
- Increased plasma renin activity
- Increased plasma angiotensin II and plasma aldosterone
- Increased plasma vasopressin
- Decreased responsiveness to atrial natriuretic peptide

The levels of these hormones correlate with the mortality rate in heart failure and are higher in patients with symptoms who require pharmacologic treatment. How-

ever, neuroendocrine activation occurs before the onset of overt symptoms and is therefore an important
marker for patients at increased risk. In this section,
the significance of each of these hormones in heart
failure is reviewed.

Renin-Angiotensin-Aldosterone System

It is well established that the renin system plays a
central role in the pathophysiology and treatment of
congestive heart failure. However, the magnitude of
the renin response varies among patients. The
heterogeneity of this response has important ramifica-
tions when considering the pathophysiology and treatment in the individual patient with heart failure.

Cody et al demonstrated that, in patients with
symptomatic heart failure who were studied during
changes in sodium balance, the response of the renin
system paralleled that of normal individuals (Figure
6.1). Accordingly, during dietary sodium restriction
(Na = 10 mEq/d), all patients had significantly higher
PRA and urinary aldosterone excretion than on a
higher intake (Na = 100 mEq/d). These findings
illustrate that, in congestive heart failure as in normal
man, renin secretion is determined by macula densa
sodium chloride delivery and that renin activity is the
primary determinant of aldosterone excretion. Further, the study showed that a modest increase in salt
intake could markedly suppress renin and aldosterone
levels (Figure 6.1).

Those studies also indicated that in heart failure,
vasoconstriction is maintained at a constant level by
different mechanisms during variations in dietary
sodium intake. On a low sodium diet (10 mEq/d),
systemic vascular resistance and blood pressure fell
promptly in response to inhibition of angiotensin
converting enzyme (ACEI) by captopril and was therefore angiotensin-dependent. The reactive rise in renin
induced by captopril marks the activation of renal

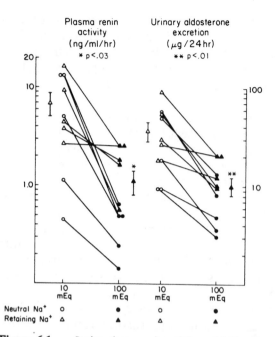

Figure 6.1 — Supine plasma renin activity and 24-h urinary aldosterone excretion for two different sodium diets. The circles represent those patients who ultimately achieved neutral sodium balance on the 100 meq sodium diet, while the triangles represent those patients who continue to retain sodium during the 100 meq sodium diet. Sodium repletion with 100 meq resulted in suppression of both plasma renin activity and urinary aldosterone secretion. However, the greatest suppression of the renin-angiotensin system during the 100 meq sodium diet was achieved in those patients who were in neutral sodium balance (closed circles). Mean values are given, ± SEM.

Reproduced from the Journal of Clinical Investigation 1986;77:1443 by copyright permission of the American Society for Clinical Investigation.

baroreceptor and macula densa signals that is characteristic of clinical states associated with angiotensin-dependent vasoconstriction (ie, renovascular hypertension). On a higher sodium intake (100 mEq/d), the level of vasoconstriction was similar to that during low sodium intake, but did not change after ACEI and was therefore angiotensin-independent.

Further assessments of the renin system in patients with severe heart failure show that during sodium repletion, two distinctly different patterns of renin system responses can occur. Approximately 50% of patients failed to achieve neutral sodium balance (where output equals intake) but, instead, avidly retained sodium and water on the 100 mEq sodium diet. Compared to the group in neutral balance, the patients that retained sodium had higher PRA and aldosterone excretion while on the higher sodium intake. Glomerular filtration rate, as estimated by creatinine clearance was similar in these two groups, although blood urea nitrogen (BUN) was significantly higher in the patients that continued to retain sodium abnormally. However, there were no differences in systemic hemodynamic characteristics, including cardiac index and mean arterial pressure. The failure to suppress renin secretion may reflect excess proximal sodium reabsorption with an inadequate macula densa signal.

Renin responses in heart failure have been useful in identifying patients who are most likely to have a favorable therapeutic response to ACEI. Packer et al re-evaluated patients with symptomatic heart failure (Class II-IV) and low PRA (< 2ng/mL/h) prior to and during chronic therapy with captopril. Approximately 50% of the patients in that study responded with sustained improvements in hemodynamic parameters (ie, cardiac index, systemic resistance, mean arterial pressure) and symptoms. These beneficial responses were accompanied by a 15-fold mean increase in PRA that was observed after several weeks of captopril treatment. In contrast, no significant hemodynamic or clinical improvement was reported in patients without this reactive rise in renin during chronic captopril therapy. These results suggest that magnitude of the effects of the renin-system (eg, vasoconstriction, aldosterone biosynthesis) are heterogenous among patients with heart failure. An analogous situation has been described in hypertension associated with low and normal plasma renin activities, but without heart failure, where the antihypertensive response to ACEI can vary widely between individuals. Altogether, the data show that a reactive plasma renin rise indicates that the ACE inhibitor treatment is effective and a useful clinical index.

In keeping with its central role in the pathophysiology of heart failure, the activity of the renin system is an important marker for cardiovascular risk. In the CONSENSUS-I trial, in which patients with severe heart failure were randomized to receive either placebo or enalapril, pretreatment plasma levels of angiotensin II and aldosterone were significantly higher in patients on placebo who died within six months (Table 6.1). Furthermore, in the enalapril group, a reduction in mortality was observed only in patients with pretreatment plasma angiotensin II and aldosterone levels above the median. The correlations between mortality and pretreatment plasma AII and aldosterone levels that were present in the placebo group were not found in the enalapril group. Taken together, these results suggest that mortality in severe heart failure is linked to the activation of the renin system and that interruption of this system improves survival.

The renin-angiotensin-aldosterone system plays an important role in the progressive left ventricular enlargement and dysfunction that occur after anterior wall infarction. Pfeffer et al reported that when treatment with captopril was begun within one month of infarction in patients with a low ejection fraction, left ventricular filling pressure decreased and end diastolic volume was lower than in the placebo group (Figure 6.2). In a subsequent large scale placebo-controlled study in patients with myocardial infarction and symptomatic left ventricular dysfunction, referred to as the Survival and Ventricular Enlargement Trial

TABLE 6.1 — BASELINE HORMONES AND SIX-MONTH MORTALITY – CONSENSUS PLACEBO GROUP			
Hormone	**Survivors (n = 68)**	**Deaths (n = 51)**	**p <**
Angiotensin II (pg/mL)	64 ± 9	93 ± 9	0.001
Aldosterone (pmol/L)	1,108 ± 95	1,627 ± 120	0.001
Atrial natriuretic peptide (pg/mL)	320 ± 95	520 ± 61	0.01
Norepinephrine (pg/mL)	750 ± 46	1,188 ± 106	0.001
Epinephrine (pg/mL)	119 ± 17	239 ± 39	0.05
Values for survivors and deaths are mean ± SEM			

Reproduced with permission. Hormone regulation cardiovascular function in patients with severe congestive heart failure and their relation to mortality. Circulation 1990;82:1730-1736. Copyright 1990, American Heart Association.

(SAVE), captopril decreased mortality from all causes (– 20%), including cardiovascular events (– 21%) (see Section #11, *Pharmacologic Therapy*). These benefits were present whether or not patients received β-adrenoceptor blockers or thrombolytic therapy, and suggested that ACEI leads to additional improvements in clinical outcome.

It is evident from these clinical and laboratory studies that in the volume overloaded ventricle, the renin system contributes to remodeling and dysfunction. Weber and his colleagues have extended these observations to hypertension, in which myocardial fibrosis appears to be an important determinant of

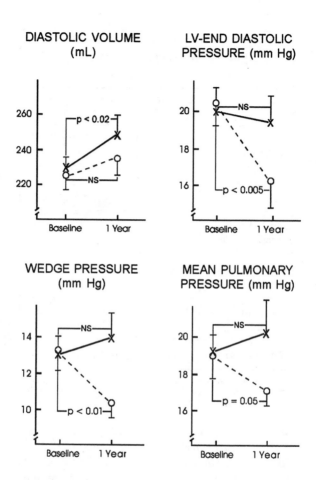

Figure 6.2 — Change in left ventricular end-diastolic pressure, pulmonary capillary wedge pressure and mean pulmonary-artery pressure between baseline and one-year evaluation in the placebo (crosses) and captopril (circles) groups.

Reprinted with permission from the New England Journal of Medicine 1988;319:83.

diastolic dysfunction. In rat models of renovascular hypertension and primary aldosteronism associated with systemic hypertension and high aldosterone levels, reactive myocardial fibrosis was not limited to the pressure overloaded left ventricle, but was also present in the right ventricle that was not exposed to a pressure load and was not hypertrophied. When hypertension was prevented by pretreatment with the aldosterone receptor antagonist spironolactone, myocardial fibrosis and ventricular hypertrophy were prevented. At lower doses that did not reduce blood pressure, myocardial fibrosis was prevented even though left ventricular hypertrophy developed. These results suggest that aldosterone excess plays an important role in the pathogenesis of myocardial fibrosis and ventricular dysfunction, and that this response may not be limited to the pressure overloaded ventricle, but may occur in other conditions associated with excess activation of the renin-angiotensin-aldosterone system.

6

Sympathetic Nervous System

Excess activation of the sympathetic nervous system is characteristic of heart failure and plasma norepinephrine levels are highly correlated with the magnitude of ventricular dysfunction and mortality (Figure 6.3). Increased sympathetic nerve activity directly promotes sodium and water retention through α-adrenoceptor-mediated vasoconstriction and tubular reabsorption and also, indirectly, by stimulating renin secretion from juxtaglomerular cells. Dietary sodium restriction and diuretic therapy produces additional increases in sympathetic activity, which can be manifested by marked stimulation of the renin system and the related angiotensin and catecholamine-mediated renal vasoconstriction. This counterregulatory response accounts, in part, for the prerenal azotemia that develops during diuretic therapy in severe heart fail-

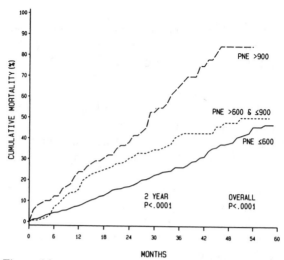

Figure 6.3 — Influence of baseline plasma norepinephrine (PNE) values on cumulative mortality. PNE levels have been divided into strata according to previous data relating these values to mortality risk.

Reproduced with permission. Francis GS, Cohn JN, Johnson JN, et al: Plasma norepinephrine PRA and CHF in V-HeFT-II. Circulation 1993;83(suppl VI):VI-43. Copyright 1993, American Heart Association.

ure. Furthermore, the related angiotensin-dependence of glomerular filtration in this setting explains the acute deterioration in GFR that can occur during treatment with ACE inhibitors (see below).

■ Vasopressin

Hyponatremia is a common manifestation of severe heart failure and it occurs when water is retained in excess of sodium. When present, hyponatremia is an ominous sign, as it has been shown to be a powerful independent predictor of cardiovascular mortality (Figure 6.4). This unfavorable prognosis was associated with marked activation of the renin system. Lee et al reported that hyponatremia patients treated with ACE inhibitors had a significantly longer period of survival than did those treated with vasodilators that

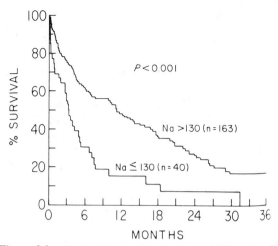

Figure 6.4 — Kaplan-Meier analysis showing cumulative rates of survival in patients with heart failure stratified into two groups based on pretreatment serum sodium concentration (> 130 vs. ≤ 130 mEq/L). Patients with severe hyponatremia had a highly unfavorable long-term prognosis (p < .001).

Reproduced with permission. Lee WH, Packer M: Prognostic importance of serum sodium concentration and its modification by converting enzyme inhibition in patients with severe chronic heart failure. Circulation 1986;73:257-269. Copyright 1986, American Heart Association.

6

did not inhibit the formation of angiotensin II. In contrast there was no selective benefit of ACEI in heart failure patients with normal serum sodium concentration in whom PRA was low or normal.

Excretion of hypoosmolar urine requires adequate delivery of filtrate to the loop of Henle and appropriate suppression of AVP secretion. Evidence points to a primary role for nonosmotic stimulation of AVP and its antidiuretic action in the development and maintenance of hyponatremia in heart failure. First, AVP levels are elevated in hyponatremia patients with heart failure whether or not they have been treated with diuretics. Secondly, in several animal models of heart failure, hyponatremia was prevented by removing the pituitary source of AVP or by treatment with an AVP antagonist.

Nonosmotic stimulation of AVP in heart failure has been related to the low stroke volume and cardiac output. Improvement in cardiac performance by afterload reduction in hyponatremia patients with heart failure decreases AVP levels and enhances water excretion. A direct effect of angiotensin II on ADH secretion has been demonstrated and therefore may provide a link between decreased cardiac performance and increased ADH secretion. Although the specific role of renin in the regulation of water balance in heart failure has not been established, it is clear that hypo-natremia is a useful clinical marker for neurohumoral activation.

■ Atrial Natriuretic Peptide

Atrial natriuretic peptide (ANP) is a vasoactive natriuretic hormone synthesized primarily by the atria in response to stretch, such as that which occurs during physiologic levels of volume expansion (Figure 6.5). There are two types of ANP receptors. The biologic receptor mediates the actions of ANP through activation of membrane-associated guanylate cyclase and the second messenger cGMP. The clearance receptor is far more abundant and is not associated with cGMP. Its main role is in the regulation of circulating levels of ANP.

The natriuretic action of ANP is the consequence of increases in GFR and a direct effect on the inner medullary collecting duct. ANP can increase GFR independent from RBF as a result of simultaneous:

- Afferent arteriolar vasodilatation
- Efferent arteriolar constriction
- Increases in K_f

This accounts for the associated increase in filtration fraction. In addition, ANP dilates vessels that have been preconstructed by:

- Norepinephrine

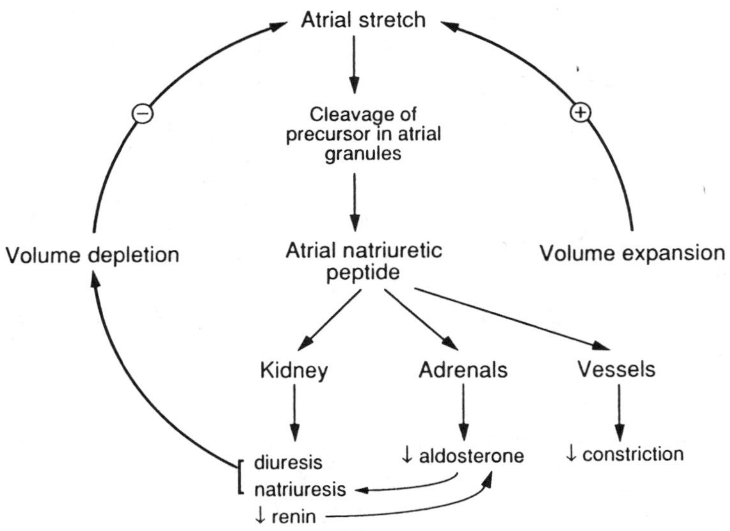

Figure 6.5 — Regulation of ANP secretion and major sites of action. Action on the kidney causes immediate salt and water excretion. Adrenal mechanism effects a delayed but more sustained increase in salt and water excretion.

Reprinted with permission. Schrier RW, Gottschalk CW: Diseases of the Kidney, 5th edition, Volume I;295. Little, Brown and Company, Copyright 1993.

- Angiotensin II (AII)
- Vasopressin
- Other agents (ie, ouabain)

Redistribution of intrarenal blood flow to the medulla may also contribute to solute washout, although a direct effect of ANP on inner medullary collecting ducts to decrease sodium reabsorption may also contribute to this response.

ANP also exerts its natriuretic action by suppressing renin secretion. This action is partly the result of the increased filtered load of sodium and chloride reaching the macula densa. Renin secretion is also inhibited *in vitro* when cGMP levels in juxtaglomerular cells are increased by ANP. Furthermore, ANP selectively reduces basal secretion of aldosterone and blocks aldosterone secretion induced by AII, but it has no effect on cortisol production.

Levels of ANP and its second messenger cGMP are increased in heart failure. However, the renal responses to ANP, including urinary sodium excretion, are attenuated in severe heart failure (Figure 6.6). Nevertheless, some studies suggest that despite the kidney's refractoriness to ANP, many extra renal responses are preserved. Specifically, ANP infusion lowers plasma aldosterone in human heart failure, despite persistently elevated plasma renin activity. Also, short-term infusions have been shown to decrease systemic vascular resistance and cardiac preload, as well as to raise cardiac output both in clinical and experimental heart failure. Thus, the preservation of these extrarenal actions suggests that increased ANP secretion by the failing heart could provide a compensatory mechanism that, to some extent, mitigates against circulatory overload.

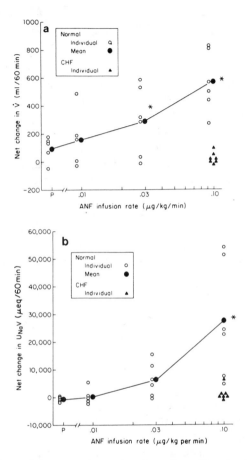

Figure 6.6 — Net changes in urine volume (V) and sodium excretion ($U_{Na}V$) during the 60-min experimental infusion phase, related to ANF infusion rate are impaired in CHF. For the normal subjects, individual values (o) and mean values (•) are given for placebo (P) and ANF infusion groups. The asterisks indicate that total excretion during ANF infusion was significantly ($p < 0.05$) greater than total excretion during the respective baseline phase. (▲) Individual responses of congestive heart failure patients to ANF infusion.

Reproduced from the Journal of Clinical Investigation, 1986;78:1362-1374 by copyright permission of the American Society for Clinical Investigation.

Endothelium-Dependent Factors

■ **Endothelin**

Endothelin (ET-1) is a potent vasoconstrictor expressed by human endothelial cells. Specific receptors are present on vascular smooth muscle, adrenal glomerulosa cells, glomeruli and papillary epithelium. ET-1 infusion results in an initial transient vasodilatation and decrease in blood pressure that may be mediated by the related increases in endothelium derived relaxing factor (EDRF) and ANP release. This is followed by a sustained increase in peripheral vascular resistance that is particularly evident in the kidney. Decreases in RBF, GFR and K_f have been reported during ET-1 administration. However, doses of ET-1 that do not impair GFR can cause natriuresis, perhaps reflecting:

- The direct effect of Na-K-ATPase inhibition by the inner medullary collecting duct epithelial cells
- Augmented ANP release, or
- The pressure natriuresis that accompanies the increase in systemic blood pressure

This effect is complimented by ET-1 attenuation of AVP-stimulated water reabsorption by the cortical collecting tubule.

Endothelin-stimulated vasoconstriction is mediated through a dose-dependent increase in cytosolic calcium which is induced by the activation of phospholipase C and phosphoinositide metabolism. The initial rise is independent from extracellular calcium, but the subsequent prolonged increase in cytoplasmic calcium is attenuated by dihydropyridine calcium channel antagonists (ie, nifedipine).

Plasma ET-1 levels were reported to be three-fold higher in patients with symptomatic heart failure as compared to normal subjects (Figure 6.7). The mag-

90

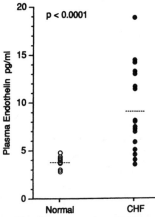

Figure 6.7 — Plot shows comparison of plasma immunoreactive endothelin-1 in normal subjects (n=12) and congestive heart failure (CHF) patients (n=20). There was a threefold increase of mean endothelin-1 values in CHF subjects compared with normal subjects (p < 0.0001).

Reproduced with permission. Luscher TF, Noll G: Endothelium-dependent vasomotion in aging, hypertension and heart failure. Circulation 1993;87(suppl VII):VII-101. Copyright 1993, American Heart Association.

nitude of the ET-1 level was directly related to the degree of pulmonary hypertension. However, the integrated effects of ET-1 on sodium and water metabolism in heart failure has not been defined.

■ Nitric Oxide

Nitric oxide (NO) is an endogenous nitrovasodilator formed in the endothelium by the conversion of arginine to citrulline. This reaction is catalyzed by a constituitive calcium-dependent enzyme, NO synthase. Inhibition of this enzyme *in vivo* by analogues of L-arginine (ie, N^G-monomethyl-L-arginine) causes vasoconstriction, suggesting that the circulation is in a state of vasodilatation that is NO-dependent. NO formation can be stimulated by:

- Shear stress related to blood flow

- Specific receptor activation mediated by:
  - Acetylcholine
  - Bradykinin
  - Platelet-derived products
  - Others

Cyclic GMP, formed in vascular smooth muscle, is the second messenger responsible for NO-mediated vasodilatation. A second form of NO synthase is present in vascular smooth muscle, where it is induced by interleukin-1 during septic shock.

In patients with heart failure, the stimulated release of NO mediated by muscarinic receptors (eg, acetylcholine) are attenuated in peripheral and coronary circulations (Figure 6.8). In contrast, endothelium-dependent relaxation in response to α_2- agonists is preserved in experimental models.

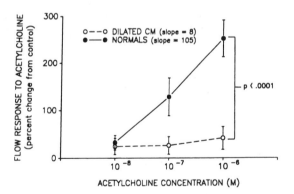

Figure 6.8 — Plot of coronary flow response to serial infusions of acetylcholine expressed as percentage of change from baseline flow. Flow response to acetylcholine was greater in control patients than in patients with dilated cardiomyopathy (CM). P value refers to comparison of slopes; error bars represent ± SEM values.

Reproduced with permission. Luschen TF, Noll G: Endothelium-dependent vasomotion in aging, hypertension and heart failure. Circulation 1993;87(suppl VII):VII-100. Copyright 1993, American Heart Association.

Integrated Renal Responses to Neuroendocrine Activation

As cardiac output decreases, renin secretion increases in response to signals from baroreceptors and the macula densa integrated at the juxtaglomerular apparatus (Figure 6.9). Increasing circulating levels of angiotensin II and catecholamines initially preserve GFR by maintaining glomerular ultrafiltration pressure through efferent arteriolar vasoconstriction. However, RBF decreases in response to the increase in renal vascular resistance. The rise in filtration fraction promotes peritubular capillary hemodynamic changes that favor proximal sodium and water reabsorption. In addition, sodium reabsorption by distal nephron segments is increased in response to elevated levels of aldosterone and AVP. The nonosmotic stimulation of AVP also impairs excretion of free water, leading to hyponatremia.

As heart failure progresses and afferent and efferent arteriolar vasoconstriction increases, filtration pressure equilibrium may be reached and GFR becomes directly dependent upon RBF. This occurs more frequently in older patients, in whom RBF is lower. In addition, K_f, and thus GFR, decrease in response to high circulating levels of AII, ADH and epinephrine.

The renal hemodynamic and excretory effects of neurohumoral activation are apparent during pharmacologic interventions. For example, ACE inhibitors improve cardiac output, RBF and GFR by interrupting AII formation. Furthermore, ACE inhibitors promote sodium and water excretion by decreasing aldosterone and AVP release. However, ACEI can cause hypotension and acute renal failure in patients with severe cardiac dysfunction in whom blood pressure and renal function are high, dependent upon AII-

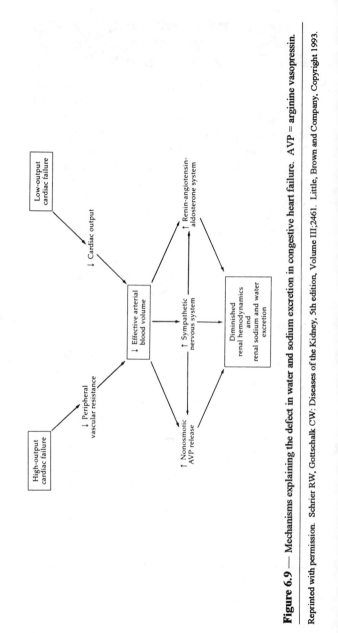

Figure 6.9 — Mechanisms explaining the defect in water and sodium excretion in congestive heart failure. AVP = arginine vasopressin.

Reprinted with permission. Schrier RW, Gottschalk CW: Diseases of the Kidney, 5th edition, Volume III;2461. Little, Brown and Company, Copyright 1993.

mediated vasoconstriction. Furthermore, non-steroidal anti-inflammatory agents, by inhibiting synthesis of vasodilating prostaglandins, can also cause acute renal failure in this setting. Patients at risk for these adverse responses have clinical evidence for neurohumoral activation and can often be identified by:

- Prerenal azotemia
- Hyponatremia
- High PRA

REFERENCES

1. Rose BD: Regulation of the effective circulating volume. In: Clinical Physiology of Acid-base and Electrolyte Disorders, 3rd edition. Rose BD (ed). New York: McGraw-Hill, 1989.

2. Schrier RW: Pathogenesis of sodium and water retention in high-output and low-output cardiac failure, nephrotic syndrome, cirrhosis and pregnancy. New Engl J Med 1988;319:1065-1127.

3. Humes HD, Gottlieb MN, Brenner BM: The kidney in congestive heart failure: with emphasis on the role of the renal microcirculation in the pathogenesis of sodium retention. In: Sodium and Water Homeostasis. Brenner BM, Stein JH (eds). New York: Churchill Livingstone, 1978;1:51-72.

4. Rabkin R, Dahl D: Hormones and the kidney. In: Diseases of the Kidney, 5th edition. Schrier RW, Gottschalk CW (eds). Boston: Little, Brown and Company, 1993;chapter 9.

5. Bichet DG, Schrier RW: Cardiac failure, liver disease and nephrotic syndrome. In: Diseases of the Kidney, 5th edition. Schrier RW, Gottschalk CW (eds). Boston: Little, Brown and Company, 1993;chapter 90.

6. Cody RJ, et al: Sodium and water balance in chronic congestive heart failure. J Clin Invest 1986;77:1441-1452.

7. Packer M, Medina N, Yushak M: Efficacy of captopril in low-renin congestive heart failure. Importance of sustained reactive hyperreninemia in distinguishing responders from nonresponders. Am J Cardiol 1984;54:771-777.

6

8. Francis GS, et al: Comparison of neuroendocrine activation in patients with and without congestive heart failure. Circulation 1990;82:1724-1729.

9. Swedberg K, et al: Hormones regulating cardiovascular function in patients with severe congestive heart failure and their relation to mortality. Circulation 1990;82:1730-1736.

10. Pfeffer MA, et al: Effect of captopril on mortality and morbidity in patients with left ventricular dysfunction after myocardial infarction. N Engl J Med 1992;327:669-677.

11. Lee WH, Packer M: Prognostic importance of serum sodium concentration and its modification by converting enzyme inhibition in patients with severe congestive heart failure. Circulation 1986;73:257-267.

12. Cody RJ, et al: Regulation of glomerular filtration in chronic congestive heart failure patients. Kidney Int 1988;34:361-367.

13. Cody RJ, et al: Atrial natriuretic factor in normal subjects and heart failure patients. J Clin Invest 1986;78:1362-1374.

14. Laragh JH: Atrial natriuretic hormone and the renin-aldosterone axis and blood pressure-electrolyte homeostasis. New Engl J Med 1985;313:1330-1340.

15. Ballermann BJ, et al: Vasoactive peptides and the kidney. In: The Kidney, 4th edition. Brenner BM, Rector FC (eds). Philadelphia: WB Saunders, 1991;chapter 14.

16. Luscher TF, Noll G: Endothelium-dependent vasomotion in aging, hypertension and heart failure. Circulation 1993;87(suppl VII):VII-97–VII-103.

17. Dzau VJ, et al: Prostaglandins in severe congestive heart failure: relation to activation of the renin-angiotensin-aldosterone system and hyponatremia. N Engl J Med 1984;310:347-352.

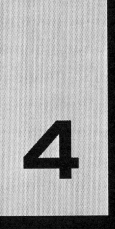

PART 4

DIAGNOSING
HEART FAILURE

7   The Clinical History

Diagnosing heart failure is a relatively straight forward process although the heart itself produces no clinical symptoms when it fails as a pump. Symptoms will be found instead in derangements of the:

- Lungs
- Kidneys
- Liver
- Other organs

The clinician will use the following steps in identifying the heart failure syndrome:

- A complete patient history
- Physical examination
- Routine laboratory tests

The New York Heart Association (NYHA) functional classification of heart failure is a standard method of assessing clinical status:

Class I   No limitation of physical activity; no dyspnea, fatigue or palpitations with ordinary physical activity

Class II   Slight limitation of activity; patients have fatigue, palpitations and dyspnea with ordinary physical activity, but are comfortable at rest

Class III   Marked limitation of activity; less than ordinary physical activity results in symptoms, but patients are comfortable at rest

Class IV   Symptoms are present at rest and they are exacerbated by any physical exertion

More advanced heart failure, as determined by NYHA functional class, is associated with decreased survival. However, patients become symptomatic only after marked deterioration of myocardial function and so this is an insensitive diagnostic tool (see Section #9, *Laboratory and Imaging Studies*).

Left and Right Ventricular Failure

Forward and backward heart failure are terms with some limited usefulness in describing and loosely distinguishing clinical signs and symptoms. Forward failure generally implies that the patient's symptoms and signs stem from a low cardiac output resulting in:
- Fatigability
- Weakness
- Mental confusion
- Possibly oliguria
- Even shock

Backward failure generally implies that pulmonary or systemic venous congestion are the consequence of elevated venous pressure behind the failing ventricles, either because of:
- Myocardial dysfunction, or
- Valvular abnormalities

Left-heart failure indicates that the primary impairment is of the left side of the heart while right-heart failure implicates the right side. However, both sides of the heart function in series unless there are shunts or regurgitant valves. Therefore, neither side of the heart can pump significantly more blood than the other. In time, the failure of one side affects the other – if the output of one side decreases, the input and thus the output of the other will also decrease. Thus, the most common origin of right-heart failure is left-heart failure.

Dyspnea

"Shortness of breath" on exertion is the most common patient complaint and generally comes early in the development of left-heart failure. It is caused by elevated left atrial, pulmonary venous and pulmonary capillary pressures, and engorgement of the pulmonary capillary-venous bed (Figure 7.1); this brings about reduced pulmonary compliance and increases the work of breathing, particularly when physical effort amplifies cardiac output.

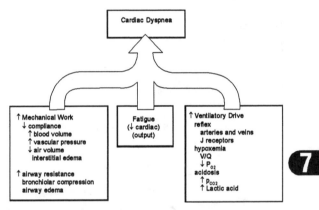

Figure 7.1 — Factors that induce an increase in mechanical work of ventilation and ventilatory drive in states of pulmonary venous hypertension resulting from increased left heart filling pressure. The simultaneous occurrence of these factors and muscular fatigue converge to produce the sensation of dyspnea.

Turino GM: Origins of cardiac dyspnea. Primary Cardiology 1981;7:76. Reprinted with permission.

It should be kept in mind that some patients may not report dyspnea on exertion simply because they do not exert themselves, being bedridden or completely sedentary. Also, the dyspnea of congestive heart failure must be distinguished from that resulting from other disorders (Table 7.1). While the development of

101

TABLE 7.1 — NONCARDIAC CAUSES OF PULMONARY EDEMA

Decreased plasma oncotic pressure:
- Hypoalbuminemia due to:
  - Renal disease
  - Hepatic disease
  - Nutritional cause
  - Protein-losing enteropathy

Altered alveolar-capillary membrane permeability (adult respiratory distress syndrome)
- Pneumonia:
  - Viral
  - Bacterial
  - Parasitic
  - Aspiration
- Inhaled toxins:
  - Smoke
  - Nitrogen dioxide
  - Phosgene
- Circulating toxins:
  - Bacterial endotoxins
  - Snake venom
- Radiation pneumonia
- Endogenous vasoactive substances:
  - Kinins
  - Histamines
- Disseminated intravascular coagulation
- Uremia
- Immunologic reactions (hypersensitivity pneumonitis)
- Drowning

Lymphatic insufficiency:
- Carcinomatosis
- Fibrosing lymphangitis

Unknown or not well understood:
- Narcotic overdose (heroin)
- High altitude pulmonary edema
- Neurogenic:
  - Subarachnoid hemorrhage
  - Central nervous system trauma
- Eclampsia
- Post-cardiopulmonary bypass
- Post-cardioversion
- Post-anesthesia
- Pheochromocytoma

From: Kloner RA, Dzau VJ: Heart Failure. In: The Guide to Cardiology, 2nd edition. Kloner RA (ed). New York: LeJacq Communications, 1990;chapter 23. Reprinted with permission.

dyspnea over a short period of time is characteristic of heart failure, a more gradual process suggests primary pulmonary disease. Patients with anxiety-based dyspnea tend to manifest slow and profound sighing and hyperventilation, in contrast to the fast and shallow breathing pattern more typical of heart failure.

Orthopnea

The patient with orthopnea experiences labored breathing when lying relatively flat in bed and finds relief by assuming a more upright position. The upright position lowers the diaphragm, increasing ventilatory reserve while the gravitational effect relieves venous return and pulmonary hydrostatic pressure. In the heart failure syndrome, orthopnea usually manifests later than exertional dyspnea. The heart failure patient with orthopnea characteristically requires several pillows in order to sleep in relative comfort. However, the physician must elicit the information, not usually volunteered, that the need for pillows represents a distinct change before concluding that the phenomenon is due to heart failure.

Paroxysmal Nocturnal Dyspnea

In this terrifying symptom, the patient awakens suddenly, feeling suffocated, a few hours after retiring. Relief comes after sitting on the edge of the bed awhile, coughing or gasping, or going to the window for fresh air. The mechanisms responsible for such an attack of dyspnea are similar to those for orthopnea, and represent markedly impaired cardiac function.

It should be noted that paroxysmal nocturnal dyspnea, brought on by increasing wheezing and accumulations of secretions when lying flat, can also occur in patients with advanced chronic obstructive pulmonary disease. A similar symptom, associated with hyperventilation, may occur in patients with a history of anxiety.

Cheyne-Stokes Respiration

Cheyne-Stokes respiration, consisting of alternating periods of apnea and hyperpnea, and considered to be a dominant symptom of left-heart failure, tends to occur soon after the patient goes to sleep. Typically, the patient awakens during the rapid phase that follows the period of apnea. The phenomenon is intensified by sedatives or opiates.

Acute Pulmonary Edema

Patients with acute pulmonary edema, usually terrified, remain upright if they are able. They are:
- Anxious
- Agitated
- Pale
- Sweaty
- Skin tends to be:
  - Cold
  - Clammy
  - Cyanotic

The respiratory rate is rapid (30 to 40 per minute) while the depth of respiration can be either deep or shallow. Nostrils are flared, accessory respiratory muscles may be used, and the intercostal supraclavicular areas tend to be retracted. They may cough, wheeze and exhibit tracheal rattling sounds. Sputum may be profuse, brothy or tinged with blood. The pulse is also rapid – if it is not, heart block should be suspected. Systolic and diastolic blood pressures may be elevated even in the absence of prior hypertension; low blood pressure indicates cardiogenic shock. Systemic venous pressure is usually elevated. Bubbling rales, wheezing and rhonchi may be heard, obscuring the heart sounds.

If the patient is too ill to provide a history and the heart sounds are obscured by wheezing, it may be difficult to distinguish acute pulmonary edema from asthma. A chest x-ray will usually yield the proper diagnosis, and until then it would be wiser to rely on the following:

- Aminophylline
- Oxygen
- Intravenous diuretic
- Sublingual or intravenous nitroglycerin

Nocturnal Cough

An unproductive cough, with or without rales, particularly bothersome during the night, may also be due to chronic heart failure. Angiotensin converting enzyme inhibitors can produce a similar type of nocturnal cough. However, additional history, physical signs and appropriate diagnostic studies can usually distinguish these causes.

Hemoptysis

The patient with chronic congestive heart failure may complain of streaks of blood in the sputum caused by alveolar hemorrhage. However, other causes of hemoptysis should be considered, including pulmonary infarction or malignancy, and chronic bronchitis.

Unexplained Weight Gain

The abnormal retention of sodium and water that is characteristic of chronic heart disease can be reflected in unexplained weight gain. Loss of five pounds or more in 24 to 36 hours after administration of a diuretic confirms this as the cause.

Edema becomes clinically evident only after approximately five liters of fluid has been retained. Although some patients may gain 10 pounds or more without developing peripheral edema, most will note that by evening their feet are swollen and that the skin above the sock line is pitted or depressed. In the case of the patient who has been in bed for several days, fluid accumulation may be absent in the lower extremities, appearing instead in the scrotal and lumbosacral area and, in the most severe cases, over most of the body including the chest. Such dependent edema in the early course of congestive heart disease is virtually always associated with elevated central venous pressure (see Section #8, *Central Venous Pressure*); if central venous pressure is not abnormally high other causes of edema should be explored.

Other, noncardiac causes of peripheral edema are:
- Varicose veins
- Obesity
- Phlebitis
- Pregnancy
- Liver disease
- Renal disease
- Cyclic edema
- Corticosteroid or vasodilator administration
- Retroperitoneal tumor
- Even prolonged periods of standing or sitting

Nocturia

This occurs relatively early in the course of heart failure. Urine output decreases when upright because of increased systemic vascular resistance. When recumbent, venous return increases, renal vasoconstriction decreases, and urine output increases.

Increasing Body Girth

Ascites is more prone to occur in patients with heart failure who also have:
- Cirrhosis
- Constrictive pericarditis
- Restrictive cardiomyopathy
- Tricuspid valve disease

A marked increase in body girth may be a clue to this condition.

Weakness

Weakness and fatigue can be prominent symptoms in patients with advanced heart failure. This may arise from inadequate blood flow to skeletal muscle during:
- Exertion
- Potassium depletion
- Anorexia caused by drug toxicity or progressive heart failure

Weakness, exhaustion and postural hypotension can follow excessive diuresis with an associated fall in cardiac output.

Mental Symptoms

Some patients with congestive heart failure may manifest emotional disorders stemming from their perception of their illness and the limited activity it imposes. As heart failure progresses and cardiac output declines, impaired cerebral blood flow may lead to:
- Dizziness
- Sleepiness
- Confusion

Gastrointestinal Symptoms

Patients with congestive heart disease may report:
- Anorexia
- Nausea
- Vomiting
- Abdominal distension
- Constipation
- Abdominal pain

The cause of these symptoms may lie in venous engorgement and congestion of the gastrointestinal tract or to digoxin toxicity. In severe heart failure, intense splanchnic vasoconstriction may even lead to intestinal ischemia.

Pain and tenderness in the right upper quadrant and hepatic pain on effort may occur, as a result of tension on the liver capsule caused by engorgement and congestion.

Cachexia

Cachexia may be marked in the late stages of congestive heart failure, brought about by:
- Hypermetabolism
- Protein-losing enteropathy
- Poor appetite resulting from congestion
- Drug toxicity
- Mental depression
- Hypoxia

Tumor necrosis factor is elevated in severe heart failure and may contribute to this condition.

Cyanosis

Although arterial oxygen saturation may be normal, the oxygen content of the venous blood may be decreased because of increased oxygen extraction by tissues receiving a low blood flow. This may result in a "dusky" cast on the faces and distal extremities of patients with severe heart failure.

Review

Major clinical symptoms of left-heart failure are:
- Exertional dyspnea
- Orthopnea
- Paroxysmal nocturnal dyspnea
- Dyspnea at rest
- Exercise intolerance
- Weakness
- Fatigue
- Nocturia
- Mental confusion

Major clinical symptoms of right-heart failure are:
- Systemic venous congestion including dependent edema
- Right upper quadrant pain due to stretching of the hepatic capsule from liver engorgement
- Anorexia
- Nausea
- Bloating, due to congestion of the mesentery and liver
- Fatigue
- Unlikely pulmonary symptoms unless left-heart failure is also present

REFERENCES

1. Ghali JK, et al: Precipitating factors leading to decompensation of heart failure. Arch Intern Med 1988;148:1290-1295.

2. Kloner RA, Dzau VG: Heart failure. In: The Guide to Cardiology, 2nd edition. Kloner RA (ed). New York: Le Jacq Communications, 1990;359-382.

3. Perloff JK: The clinical manifestations of cardiac failure in adults. In: The Myocardium: Failure and Infarction. Braunwald E (ed). New York: HP Publishing Co, Inc., 1974;93-100.

4. Rapaport E: Congestive heart failure: diagnosis and principles of treatment. In: Drug Treatment of Heart Failure. Cohn JN (ed). New York: Yorke Medical Books, 1983;73-89.

5. Levine B, et al: Elevated circulating levels of tumor necrosis factor in severe chronic heart failure. N Engl J Med 1990;323:236-241.

8   The Physical Examination

General Appearance

In the earlier stages of congestive heart disease, dyspnea is apparent only after mild exertion. In the later stages, respiratory distress may be evident even at rest. Tachycardia at rest with or without reduced pulse and premature ventricular beats may be noted. Cachexia can be extreme in the advanced stages; it is the result of:

- Hypermetabolism
- Protein-losing enteropathy
- Poor appetite because of congestion
- Drug toxicity
- Mental depression
- Cellular hypoxia

It must be kept in mind that signs and symptoms of peripheral or circulatory congestion do not always signify congestive heart disease. Congestive heart failure is not usually present if the ECG is normal and the heart is not enlarged. For example, circulatory congestion can occur postoperatively in patients who have received large amounts of blood and fluids: their symptoms arise from hypervolemia. The telling clue is that these patients respond to the increase in filling pressure with increased systolic function. This may reflect impaired renal excretory function caused by renal parenchymal disease or bilateral renal artery stenosis. Furthermore, when there is marked peripheral edema and low or normal central filling pressures, the cause of circulatory congestion should be sought in such extracardiac origins as cirrhosis.

In the overwhelming majority of patients with heart failure, the heart is enlarged. Exceptions to this include:

- Constrictive pericarditis
- Restrictive myocardial disease
- Acute decompensation following myocardial infarction

The enlargement may be either in the ventricle or atrium or in both, driven by increasing filling pressures. While the enlargement may be apparent in the chest x-ray, it can also be noted in the physical examination. The apical impulse is displaced laterally or downward, and if it has a thrusting quality, pronounced left ventricular activity can be assumed.

The S_3-gallop is recognized to be the hallmark of left ventricular failure. This sound, best heard with light pressure over the left ventricular apex, occurs in early diastole, reflecting rapid ventricular filling into a noncompliant or overly distended ventricle. However, it can also be heard, in the absence of heart failure, in:

- Healthy children and adolescents
- Pregnancy
- Mitral regurgitation
- Tricuspid regurgitation
- Patent ductus arteriosus
- Interventricular septal defect
- Interatrial septal defect

An S_4-gallop, while generally reflecting decreased left ventricular function, may also be heard. However, by itself it does not necessarily indicate heart failure. With a very rapid heart rate, the S_3 and S_4 may merge into a single loud gallop in mid-diastole.

Soft apical murmurs reflecting mitral or tricuspid insufficiency are not reliable in establishing a diagnosis of heart failure. A surer but less common sign is *pulsus alternans*, the initial variations in Korotkoff sounds that are heard as cuff pressure is slowly lowered. This phenomenon is indicative of severe left ventricular failure.

Lungs

Transudation of fluid into interstitial and interalveolar space occurs as a consequence of elevated pulmonary capillary pressure. The first auscultatory sign is fine rales at the dependent, posterior lung bases. As heart failure progresses, the rales become more widely distributed over the entire chest and are more coarse and moist, even to the extent of obscuring the breath sounds. Edema of the bronchial walls may cause bronchospasm, manifested as wheezing and expiratory rhonchi. However, it is important to recognize that:

- Heart failure often occurs without the development of pulmonary rales
- Rales may be due to noncardiac disease

8

Central Venous Pressure

Elevated central venous pressure, indicating decompensating heart failure, can be assessed by an examination of the deep jugular veins. With the patient propped in bed at a 45° angle, the peak of the maximum venous pulsation should not rise more than the normal 2 cm above the sternal angle. In extremely severe heart failure it may be necessary to make this examination with the patient sitting at an angle of 90°. If 5 cm (the putative vertical distance between the sternal angle and the midline of the right atrium) is added to the above estimation, the hydrostatic level of the central venous pressure and the right ventricular end-diastolic pressure may be stated: 7 cm is normal.

At times it is not possible to achieve an unequivocal determination by the above maneuver. In this case the physician should compare the normal central venous pressure with that resulting from a test for hepatojugular reflux. In this test, with the patient at a 45° angle and instructed to keep his mouth open in order to avoid the Valsalva maneuver, the periumbilical region is compressed for 30 to 60 seconds. If peak jugular venous pressure consequently rises beyond the normal 2 cm level, it indicates that the failing heart is not able to adjust to the increased venous return induced by the compression of the liver.

Abdomen

The liver may become enlarged and tender with severe heart failure and the consequent high systemic venous pressure. The presence of ascites may be due to chronic heart failure and indicates an advanced phase. Splenomegaly often accompanies hepatomegaly and may be associated with cardiac cirrhosis.

Eyes

A staring appearance with slight exophthalmus, reflecting elevated venous pressure, may indicate long-standing severe heart failure. Occasionally, jaundice will be seen in patients with heart failure, but the bilirubin level is seldom greater than 2 mg/dl. This should suggest pulmonary infarction as well as centrilobular hepatic necrosis.

REFERENCES

1. Ghali JK, et al: Precipitating factors leading to decompensation of heart failure. Arch Intern Med 1988;148:1290-1295.

2. Kloner RA, Dzau VG: Heart failure. In: The Guide to Cardiology, 2nd edition. Kloner RA (ed). New York: LeJacq Communications, 1990;359-382.

3. Perloff JK: The clinical manifestations of cardiac failure in adults. In: The Myocardium: Failure and Infarction. Braunwald E (ed). New York: HP Publishing Co, Inc., 1974;93-100.

4. Rapaport E: Congestive heart failure: diagnosis and principles of treatment. In: Drug Treatment of Heart Failure. Cohn JN (ed). New York: Yorke Medical Books, 1983;73-89.

8

9 Laboratory and Imaging Studies

Clinical assessment of the severity of heart failure is commonly based upon limitation of exercise capacity as defined by the New York Heart Association functional classification (see Section #7, *The Clinical History*). However, patients generally remain asymptomatic until left ventricular ejection fraction and aerobic capacity have increased by 40 to 50% below normal (Figure 9.1). This finding indicates that the relationship between the severity of symptoms and the magnitude of left ventricular dysfunction is not very sensitive.

Given the high mortality rate in patients with heart failure, additional objective measurements are required to assess the extent of cardiac disease and prognosis. Clinical trials in heart failure have been demonstrated that patients at increased risk of premature death can be identified by the presence of ventricular arrhythmias and neurohumoral activation (ie, plasma norepinephrine) in addition to the level of impairment of ventricular function and exercise tolerance. The noninvasive and invasive procedures used to evaluate these determinants of risk in the heart failure patient are outlined in this section.

Electrocardiogram

There are no specific electrocardiogram (ECG) abnormalities associated with heart failure. Signs of ischemia or infarction, if present, may point to an etiology for acute or chronic heart failure. Similarly, evidence for left ventricular hypertrophy may be present in hypertension or hemodynamically advanced aortic

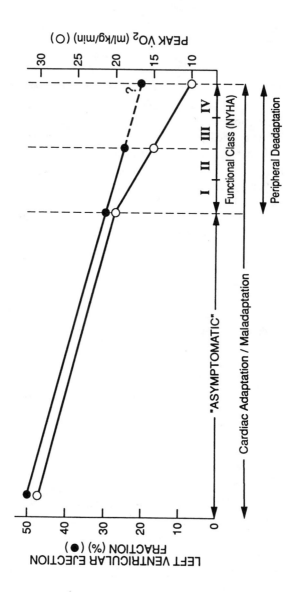

Figure 9.1 — Graph of left ventricular ejection fraction (LVEF [%]) and peak oxygen consumption (peak VO_2, $mL \cdot kg^{-1} \cdot min^{-1}$) as a function of the severity of symptoms during the course of the syndrome of congestive heart failure (CHF) as derived from data in the prevention and treatment arms of the SOLVD trials. During the so-called "asymptomatic phase" of the syndrome, LVEF decreases from a normal value of > 50% to 28%. With the development of symptoms compatible with functional Class II-III according to the New York Heart Association (NYHA), LVEF decreases only slightly further to 24%. What happens to LVEF when patients develop symptoms compatible with functional Class IV has not been studied in a large multicenter trial but can reasonably be assumed to range from 18 to 24%. Peak VO_2, ie, peak aerobic capacity, is 30 mL · $kg^{-1} \cdot min^{-1}$ for a normal subject aged 60 to 65 years. Surprisingly, so-called "asymptomatic" patients with LVEF of 28% have already experienced a substantial reduction in peak VO_2 to 20 mL · $kg^{-1} \cdot min^{-1}$. From 30 to 20 mL · $kg^{-1} \cdot min^{-1}$, the decline in peak VO_2 parallels that of LVEF, which suggests that reduced left ventricular performance plays a major role in the decrease in peak aerobic capacity. When patients develop symptoms compatible with functional Class II-III and IV, peak VO_2 declines further to 15 and 10 mL · $kg^{-1} \cdot min^{-1}$, respectively. From 20 to 10 mL · $kg^{-1} \cdot min^{-1}$, the decline in peak VO_2 is far greater than the fall in LVEF. Indeed, at this state, LVEF and VO_2 max are no longer directly related.

Reproduced with permission. LeJemtel TA, Sonnenblick EH: Heart failure: adoptive and maladoptive processes. Circulation 1993;87(suppl VII):VII-3. Copyright 1993, American Heart Association.

9

stenosis, suggesting excessive pressure loading. Left atrial enlargement may indicate the mitral valvular disease. However, echocardiography is a much more useful tool for assessing cardiac geometry and valvular integrity (see below).

Chest X-Ray

A thorough radiologic examination of the chest is an important part of the routine evaluation of the patient believed to be in heart failure. The chest x-ray allows direct observation of:

- Cardiac size
- Pulmonary parenchyma
- Vasculature

Roentgenographic evidence of cardiac enlargement occurs when the cardiothoracic ratio (CTR) exceeds 0.5, measured by dividing the maximal cardiac silhouette diameter by the maximal internal thoracic diameter.

CTR was a highly significant predictor of mortality in the Veterans Administration Vasodilator-Heart Failure Trials (Figure 9.2). There was an inverse relation between CTR and survival, where annual mortality increased at a greater rate when CTR was above 0.55. However, in those trials there was only a weak correlation between CTR and left ventricular ejection fraction and peak oxygen consumption during exercise. Therefore, CTR should not be used to predict the presence or severity of left ventricular dysfunction.

Other studies have reported that roentgenographic evidence of cardiac enlargement is particularly ominous after myocardial infarction. Survivors of myocardial infarction who developed left heart enlargement were more likely to develop angina, symptomatic heart failure and had increased mortality rates when compared to those with normal cardiac silhouettes.

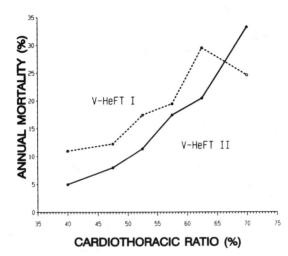

Figure 9.2 — Graph showing annual mortality rates for cardiothoracic ratio.

Reproduced with permission. Cohn JN, Johnson GR, Skabetai R: Ejection fraction, peak exercise oxygen consumption, cardiothoracic ratio, ventricular arrhythmias and plasma norepinephrine as determinants of prognosis in heart failure. Circulation 1993;83(suppl VI):VI-11. Copyright 1993, American Heart Association.

Changes in pulmonary vasculature can be observed as pulmonary capillary pressure increases. Mild increase in pressure (ie, 13 to 18 mmHg) results in equalization in the size of vessels at the apex and base of the lung. As pressures increase (ie, 18 to 23 mmHg), pulmonary vascular redistribution occurs with further filtration of apical vessels. At pressures greater than 20 mmHg, interstitial pulmonary edema occurs, with:

- Kerley B lines
- Perivascular cuffing
- Subpleural edema

Alveolar edema and pleural effusions occur when pressures exceed approximately 25 mmHg. However, these guidelines are relatively insensitive and when the diagnosis of elevated pulmonary capillary wedge pressure is in question, right heart catheterization provides a more definitive measurement (Figure 9.3).

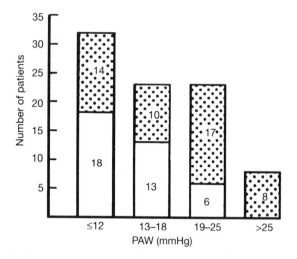

Figure 9.3 — Comparison of pulmonary artery wedge (PAW) pressure to findings of pulmonary edema in acute myocardial infarction. 14/32 patients with PAW pressures of less than 12 mmHg had findings on chest x-ray suggesting pulmonary venous hypertension (▨), and 6/23 patients with PAW wedge pressure of 10 to 25 mmHg had normal lung vasculature (☐).

Rahimtoola SH: Management of congestive heart failure. Clinical Cardiology 1992;15(suppl I):I-22–I-27. This figure was reprinted with permission of Clinical Cardiology Publishing Co., Inc.; Box 832; Mahwah, NJ 07430-0832 USA.

Echocardiography

Compared with the chest x-ray, the echocardiogram provides a more sensitive index of cardiac geometry including atrial and ventricular chamber dimensions, wall thicknesses and ventricular mass. It also provides a highly sensitive measurement of valvular structure and function which may lead to the diagnosis of surgically remediable heart failure.

The contractile state of the left ventricle can also be assessed echocardiographically. Several studies have identified echocardiographic indices which are useful in detecting severe and prognostically important abnormalities of left ventricular contractility. In the V-HeFT trials, baseline measurements of end systolic left ventricular chamber radius to wall thickness ratio (Rs:THs), left ventricular internal dimension during systole (LVIDs), and mitral E point separation (EPSS) were significant predictors of mortality. Furthermore, treatment with hydralazine and nitrates resulted in parallel improvements in both EPSS and left ventricular ejection fraction (LVEF).

These echocardiographic findings may be explained by the law of LaPlace in which wall stress is directly related to the product of pressure and radius, and indirectly related to wall thickness. Patients with a lower mass:volume ratio may not tolerate dilatation as well because of the related increase in wall stress and oxygen consumption. In addition, several studies have found an inverse relation between EPSS and LVEF.

Echocardiographic variables are useful in assessing cardiac anatomy and determining cardiovascular risk. When combined with other prognostic indicators, it is also an important tool for identifying patients with potential curable forms of heart failure.

9

Radionuclide Cineangiography

Radionuclide cineangiography (RNCA) is useful in assessing patients with symptoms suggestive of heart failure. It is a sensitive, noninvasive measure of right and left ventricular function and can distinguish global and regional abnormalities ventricular aneurysm. In addition, ischemic heart disease can be identified by an exercise-induced fall in global ejection fraction and development of regional wall abnormalities, although an abnormal response can also occur in pressure- or volume-overloaded states not associated with coronary artery disease.

Ejection fraction (EF), as determined by RNCA, is an important prognostic determinant of mortality in patients with heart failure (Figure 9.4). Mortality rates are higher in patients with lower ejection fraction and improvement in this measure of ventricular performance has been associated with improved survival.

By itself, EF is an imprecise determinant of the abnormalities that contribute to systolic dysfunction, such as alterations in contractility or loading parameters. Nevertheless, this measure of ventricular performance is valuable for monitoring the response to treatment of heart failure and is also an important index of cardiotoxicity of drugs (ie, doxorubicin) that may be used to treat noncardiac disorders.

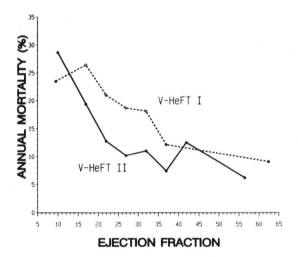

Figure 9.4 — Graph showing annual mortality rates for left ventricular ejection fraction.

Reproduced with permission. Cohn JN, Johnson GR, Skabetai R: Ejection fraction, peak exercise oxygen consumption, cardiothoracic ratio, ventricular arrhythmias and plasma norepinephrine as determinants of prognosis in heart failure. Circulation 1993;87(suppl VI):VI-10. Copyright 1993, American Heart Association.

Patients with heart failure have a high prevalence of arrhythmias and an increased incidence of sudden cardiac death. This may reflect:

- The state of ventricular dysfunction
- Myocardial ischemia
- Neurohumoral influences such as:
  - Increased sympathetic activity
  - Electrolyte abnormalities (ie, hypokalemia, hypomagnesemia) related to diuretic use
- Other contributory factors

Episodes of ventricular tachycardia and couplets, when detected by short term ambulatory ECG monitoring, identifies patients at increased risk of sudden death.

However, there is uncertainty regarding the role of routine ambulatory monitoring of patients with heart failure. This stems, in part, from reports that suggest that:

- Many of the sudden death events are not caused by ventricular arrhythmias
- Pharmacologic suppression of ambulatory ventricular arrhythmias does not prevent sudden death
- Treatment of heart failure with a regimen that includes an ACE inhibitor (but not a specific antiarrhythmic other than digoxin) can decrease ventricular ectopy and death

Thus, there is no clear indication for routine ambulatory ECG screening for arrhythmias in patients with heart failure. However, when ventricular arrhythmias are detected, attempts to improve heart failure treatment should be undertaken, including correction of electrolyte disturbances and optimizing the dose of ACE inhibitor. In patients with symptomatic ven-

9

tricular arrhythmias or sustained ventricular tachycardia, additional diagnostic evaluation and treatment may be warranted.

Markers of Neurohumoral Activation

The central role of neurohumoral activation in the pathophysiology of heart failure is outlined above (see Section #6, *Derangement of Volume Regulation in CHF*). Several clinical trials have established the prognostic importance of elevated levels of plasma renin activity, norepinephrine, atrial natriuretic peptide, and aldosterone in predicting mortality. These hormone levels, together with the serum sodium concentration, are also valuable markers for determining the likelihood of response to medical therapy.

Exercise Testing

Exercise testing has been utilized successfully in patients with heart failure to:
- Assess level of exercise tolerance
- Evaluate the magnitude of cardiac dysfunction
- Monitor the response to therapy

Peak bicycle exercise oxygen consumption relates inversely with mortality and, therefore, has prognostic significance in predicting survival (Figure 9.5). However, the correlation between this and other prognostic markers in heart failure (ie, EF, CTR, norepinephrine, plasma renin activity) is relatively weak.

Furthermore, data derived from exercise testing do not predictably reflect the extent to which exercise-related symptoms limit the performance of usual daily activities. Therefore, in the individual patient with heart failure, the role of exercise testing may be more suitable to assessing short-term response therapy rather than predicting long-term survival.

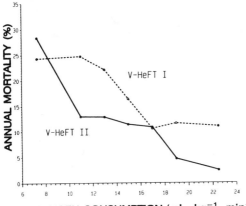

Figure 9.5 — Graph showing annual mortality rates for peak VO_2.

Reproduced with permission. Cohn JN, Johnson GR, Skabetai R: Ejection fraction, peak exercise oxygen consumption, cardiothoracic ratio, ventricular arrhythmias and plasma norepinephrine as determinants of prognosis in heart failure. Circulation 1993;87(suppl VI):VI-10. Copyright 1993, American Heart Association.

Cardiac Catheterization

Assessment of pulmonary capillary wedge pressure via a right heart catheter can provide important information regarding the initial response to treatment with afterload reducing agents. Less commonly, this method is used to distinguish between cardiac and noncardiac causes of pulmonary vascular congestion when the diagnosis cannot be established by noninvasive methods.

When ischemic heart disease is suggested by the patient's history and noninvasive assessment, coronary angiography is required to assess the severity and determine whether the lesions may be remediable by angioplasty or surgery.

Routine Laboratory Tests

As a consequence of impaired cardiac output, diminished tissue perfusion and heightened venous pressure may appear as abnormalities in routine laboratory tests. Urinalysis may show nonnephrotic range proteinuria, related to elevated angiotensin II levels or intrinsic renal parenchymal disease. Blood urea nitrogen (BUN) may be increased disproportionately to serum creatinine, and urinary specific gravity may be elevated due to prerenal azotemia and nonosmotic stimulation of ADH secretion, respectively.

Abnormalities of liver function due to passive congestion may appear as elevations of:

- Serum bilirubin
- Aspartate amino-transferase (AST)
- Serum lactic dehydrogenase (LDH)

REFERENCES

1. Cohn JN, et al: Ejection fraction, peak exercise oxygen consumption, cardiothoracic ratio, ventricular arrhythmias and plasma norepinephrine as determinants of prognosis in heart failure. Circulation 1993;87(suppl VI):VI-5–VI-16.

2. LeJemtel T, Sonnenblock EH: Heart failure: adaptive and maladaptive processes. Circulation 1993;87(suppl VII):VII-1–VII-4.

3. Pfeffer MA, Braunwald E: Ventricular remodeling after myocardial infarction: experimental observations and clinical implications. Circulations 1990;81:1161-1172.

4. Wong M, et al: Echocardiographic variables as prognostic indicators and therapeutic monitors in chronic congestive heart failure: veterans affairs cooperative studies V-HeFt-I and II. Circulation 1993;87(suppl VI):VI-65–VI-70.

5. Roman MJ, Devereux R: Comparison of noninvasive measures of contractility in dilated cardiomyopathy. Echocardiography 1991;8:139-150.

128

6. Holman BL: Nuclear cardiology. In: Heart Disease: A Textbook of Cardiovascular Medicine. Braunwald E (ed). Philadelphia: WB Saunders, 1988;chapter 11.

7. Johnson G, et al: Influence of prerandomization (baseline) variables on mortality and on the reduction of mortality by enalapril: veterans affairs cooperative studies V-HeFt-I and II. Circulation 1993;87(suppl VI):VI-32–VI-39.

8. Singh BN, et al: Prevalence, significance and control of ventricular arrhythmias. In: Heart Failure: Mechanisms and Management. Lewis BD (ed). Berlin: Springer-Verlag, 1991;346-356.

9. Francis GS, et al: Plasma norepinephrine, plasma renin activity and congestive heart failure: relations to survival and the effects of therapy in V-HeFT-II. Circulation 1993;87(suppl VI):VI-40–VI-48.

10. Wenger N: Exercise testing and training of patients with congestive heart failure and left ventricular dysfunction. In: Heart Failure: Mechanisms and Management. Lewis BD (ed). Berlin: Springer-Verlag, 1991;359-367.

11. Ziesche S, et al: Hydralazine and isosorbide dinitrate combination improves exercise tolerance in heart failure: results from V-HeFT-I and II. Circulation 1993;87(suppl VI):VI-56–VI-64.

12. Rapaport E: Congestive heart failure: diagnosis and treatment. In: Drug Treatment of Heart Failure. Cohn JN (ed). Secaucus, NJ: Advanced Therapeutics Communications, Inc., 1988;127-146.

13. Spann JF, Hurst JW: The recognition and management of congestive heart failure. In: The Heart: Arteries and Veins, 7th edition. Hurst JW, Schlant RC (eds). New York: McGraw-Hill Information Services Co., 1990;387-417.

14. Yancy CW, Firth BG: Congestive heart failure. Disease-A-Month 1988;34:469.

9

PART 5

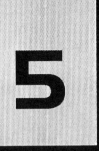

TREATMENT OF CONGESTIVE HEART FAILURE

10 Nonpharmacologic Therapy

The major goals in the management of heart failure are to improve the quality of life by relieving symptoms and to prolong life. Effective therapy should accomplish at least one of these goals. Although there can be no simple formula for treating a syndrome as variable as heart failure, certain considerations may be helpful in assessing the patient's condition that will lead to effective management. These include:

- An understanding of the nature of the underlying condition
- The rate of progression
- Associated illnesses
- Patient's age and ability to cooperate with treatment
- Response to therapy

Treatment of heart failure should be directed toward:

- Identification of correction of the underlying etiology
- Control of symptoms:
  - Nonpharmacologic treatment
  - Pharmacologic treatment
  - Cardiac transplantation

Treatment is directed against the mechanisms of congestive heart failure which have been outlined in previous sections of this book. Appropriate therapeutic strategies include:

- Controlling intravascular volume and heart rate
- Reducing impedance to left ventricular output
- Increasing myocardial contractility

Search For and Treat Underlying Causes

The search for a specific underlying cause of heart failure is the first imperative in management, and the possibility that some of such causes are correctable must be kept in mind (Table 10.1). When there is valvular insufficiency or stenosis, prosthetic valve replacement can reestablish normal or near-normal preload and afterload if myocardial contractility is reasonably intact. Similarly, surgical repair can correct such underlying mechanical origins or complications as:

- A ventricular aneurysm
- A ruptured ventricular septum
- Mitral insufficiency stemming from papillary muscle dysfunction or rupture

Myocardial revascularization may relieve the patient whose left ventricular dysfunction stems from, or is exacerbated by, myocardial ischemia.

Control of blood pressure, an important objective in any patient with hypertension, has special urgency in the management of the patient with congestive heart disease, particularly when there is myocardial damage. Since sodium accumulation and renin-mediated vasoconstriction may be factors in both hypertension and heart failure, there is considerable overlap in therapeutic strategy. The renin-sodium profile can be very useful in guiding antihypertensive therapy.

Patient Education

Among important first steps in managing congestive heart failure is educating the patient in the nature of the disease and the rationale for its therapies. A full understanding of congestive heart disease can help

TABLE 10.1 — CAUSES OF HEART FAILURE

Coronary artery disease:
- Ischemia
- Myocardial infarction
- Left ventricular aneurysm

Primary abnormality of myocardial cells:
- Cardiomyopathy
- Myocarditis

Secondary abnormality of myocardial cells:
- Prolonged hemodynamic burden (ie, primary or secondary pulmonary hypertension, polycythemia)
- Reduced O_2 delivery (ischemia)
- Toxins (eg, adriamycin)

Structural abnormalities:
- Valvular heart disease
- Pericardial disease

High-output state:
- A-V shunts (ie, cirrhosis, congenital heart disease, beri-beri)
- Anemia
- A-V fistula
- Hyperthyroidism
- Pregnancy

Other causes:
- Increased salt intake
- Inappropriate reduction of a drug regimen
- Excess exertion or emotion
- Arrhythmias
- Systemic infection
- Pulmonary embolism
- Renal failure
- Cardiac depressants (eg, disopyramide)

10

Adpated from: Kloner RA, Dzau VJ: Chapter 23: Heart Failure. In: The Guide to Cardiology, 2nd edition. Kloner RA (ed). New York: LeJacq Communications, 1990. Reprinted with permission.

dispel counterproductive fear and denial, and set the stage for compliance with treatment. Among items to be discussed in detail:

- Avoiding strenuous activity
- Maintaining an active life-style including mild exercise
- Restriction of salt intake
- Weight reduction
- Importance of compliance with medication
- Follow-up schedules

While the above nonpharmacologic measures may provide some modest therapeutic benefits in the management of congestive heart failure, their more important benefits lie in preparing the patient to play an active and cooperative role in his/her treatment, which is virtually certain to be chiefly pharmacologic.

REFERENCES

1. Cohn J: Current therapy of the failing heart. Circulation 1988;78:1099-1107.

2. Smith TW, Braunwald E, Kelly RA: Management of heart failure. In: Heart Disease: A Textbook of Cardiovascular Medicine. Braunwald E (ed). Philadelphia: WB Saunders, 1988;chapter 17.

3. Rose BD: Regulation of the effective circulating volume. In: Clinical Physiology of Acid-base and Electrolyte Disorders, 3rd edition. Rose BD (ed). New York: McGraw-Hill, 1989;chapter 17.

11   Pharmacologic Therapy

Diuretics

The central role of diuretics in the treatment of congestive heart failure indicates the importance of the kidney as the target organ of many of the hemodynamic and neurohumoral changes that occur as cardiac performance declines. Decreased cardiac output results in:

- Stimulation of the renin-angiotensin-aldosterone system
- Nonosmotic release of arginine vasopressin (AVP)
- Activation of sympathetic nervous system (SNS) with abnormal baroreceptor function and elevated plasma catecholamine levels

Renal hemodynamic changes include increased renal vascular resistance which proceeds to progressive decline in RBF and can eventually lead to impairment in GFR. Consequently, the compensatory mechanisms that maintain cardiac output and tissue perfusion by promoting sodium and water retention, also contribute to the progression of the heart failure syndrome.

The goal of diuretic therapy is to promote sodium and water excretion by the kidney. The short-term aims are to reduce cardiac filling pressure (preload) and thereby decrease congestive symptoms and decrease peripheral edema (Figure 11.1). The longer term goal is the reduction in ventricular dilatation in order to decrease ventricular wall stress.

The benefits of diuretic therapy are compromised when cardiac output falls as a result of decreased ventricular filling pressures. Patients at increased risk

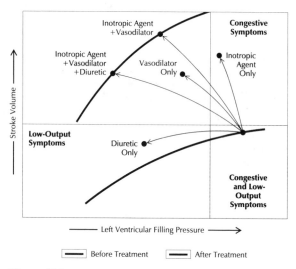

Figure 11.1 — Ventricular function curves of failing myocardium before and after treatment. Diagram predicted hemodynamic effects (and consequent impact on low-output or congestive symptoms, or both) of inotropic agents, vasodilators, and diuretics, alone or in combination. A normal ventricular function curve (omitted for clarity) would lie upward and to the left of the curves that are depicted.

Reproduced with permission. Smith TW, Kelly RA: Therapeutic strategies for CHF in the 1990s. Hospital Practice 1991;26(11):72.

for this adverse consequence are those with poor left ventricular compliance, such as concentric left ventricular hypertrophy due to aortic stenosis or hypertension. This can lead to marked neurohumoral activation in the absence of a significant reduction in systemic arterial pressure.

Several major classes of diuretics exist and they are classified according to the specific target sites on the nephron at which they impair sodium reabsorption (Figure 11.2):

- Loop diuretics in the thick ascending limb of the loop of Henle
- Thiazide-type diuretics in the distal tubule

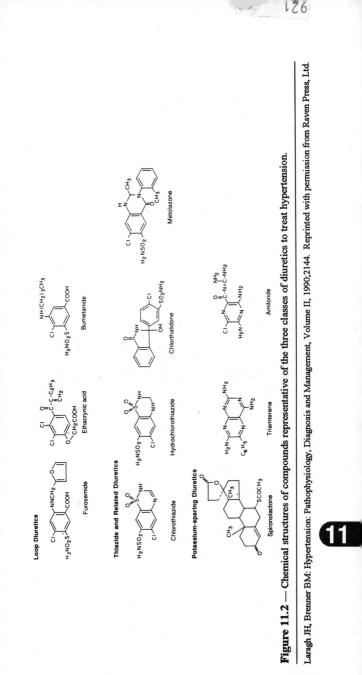

Figure 11.2 — Chemical structures of compounds representative of the three classes of diuretics to treat hypertension.

Laragh JH, Brenner BM: Hypertension: Pathophysiology, Diagnosis and Management, Volume II, 1990;2144. Reprinted with permission from Raven Press, Ltd.

- Connecting segment, potassium sparing diuretics in the aldosterone-sensitive principal cell in the cortical collecting duct (Table 11.1)
- Other minor categories include:
  - Osmotic diuretics
  - Those with actions in the proximal tubule

The potency of the diuretic is related to its site of action within the nephron. More sodium is reabsorbed in the more proximal nephron segments and, consequently, loop diuretics produce larger losses of sodium and water than do thiazide diuretics. However, diuretics with actions at the proximal tubule (ie, acetazolamide) are relatively ineffective because a large fraction of the sodium and water that exits the proximal tubule is reabsorbed at more distal segments, predominantly the loop of Henle. This attenuation of diuretic action also occurs with loop diuretics, although it is relatively minor because of the low reabsorptive capacity of the distal tubule and collecting ducts.

This section will outline the mechanisms of action of these diuretics and discuss their use in congestive heart failure (Table 11.2).

■ Loop Diuretics

The most potent diuretics used are the loop diuretics:

- Furosemide
- Bumetanide
- Ethacrynic acid

They can lead to the rapid excretion of 20 to 25% of the filtered load of sodium. They inhibit sodium reabsorption by blocking the Na-K-2Cl cotransporter in the medullary and cortical thick ascending portions of the loop of Henle, including the macula densa. The

TABLE 11.1 — Physiologic Characteristics of Commonly Used Diuretics

Site of action	Carrier or channel inhibited	Percent filtered/Na$^+$ excreted
Loop of Henle furosemide bumetanide ethacrynic acid	Na$^+$ - K$^+$ - 2Cl$^-$ carrier	up to 25%
Distal tubule and connecting system thiazides chlorthalidone metolazone	Na$^+$ - Cl$^-$ carrier	up to 3 to 5%
Cortical collecting tubule spironolactone amiloride triamterene	Na$^+$ channel	up to 1 to 2%

Rose BD: Clinical Physiology of Acid-base and Electrolyte Disorders, 3rd edition, 1989;390. Reprinted with permission from McGraw-Hill.

TABLE 11.2 — DIURETICS IN HEART FAILURE

Drugs	Site of Action	Total Daily Dose	Frequency
Acetazolamide	Proximal tubule	250 to 375 mg	qd x 2 days, skip 3rd day
Hydrochlorothiazide	Distal tubule	25 to 100 mg	qd to bid
Chlorothiazide	Distal tubule	500 to 1000 mg	qd to bid
Indapamide	Distal tubule	2.5 to 5 mg	qd
Chlorthalidone	Distal tubule	50 to 200 mg	qd
Metolazone	Distal tubule	2.5 to 10 mg	qd
Furosemide	Loop of Henle	40 to 320 mg	qd to bid
Ethacrynic Acid	Loop of Henle	50 to 400 mg	qd to bid
Bumetanide	Loop of Henle	0.5 to 10 mg	qd, bid, tid
Spironolactone (K^+-sparing)	Distal tubule	25 to 200 mg	qd to tid
Triamterene (K^+-sparing)	Distal tubule	100 to 200 mg	qd to bid
Amiloride (K^+-sparing)	Distal tubule	5 to 20 mg	qd

Reference: Physicians' Desk Reference, 48th edition. Montvale, NJ: Medical Economics Data, 1994.

cotransporter is located on the luminal surface so that higher doses are required in patients with impaired renal function.

The natriuretic response to a dose of loop diuretics is of relatively short duration, lasting approximately six hours for furosemide. During the remaining 18 hours of the day, compensatory sodium retention occurs. The mechanisms governing this antinatriuretic response are not completely understood, although it is likely due to local Starling forces favoring tubular reabsorption together with activation of the adrenergic and renin systems. This phenomenon is particularly significant in patients on high sodium intakes because the diuretic action is completely offset by the ensuing sodium retention so that by 24 hours after the dose of furosemide, no net sodium loss has occurred. This compensatory antinatriuretic effect can be overcome by maintaining a low dietary sodium intake, administering the diuretic twice daily, or, if tolerated, increasing the daily dose.

Loop diuretics can increase renal blood flow by increasing production of renal vasodilator prostaglandins and also appear to increase venous capacitance. This may account for the hemodynamic and symptomatic improvements that occur immediately after diuretic administration. Renal prostaglandins also promote sodium and water excretion. Nonsteroidal antiinflammatory agents (NSAIDs) can impair the response to diuretics and also acutely decrease RBF and GFR.

11

■ Thiazide Diuretics

Thiazide-type diuretics inhibit the Na-Cl cotransporter located at the distal tubule, and include:

- Hydrochlorothiazide
- Metolazone
- Indapamide

This nephron segment normally reabsorbs a smaller fraction of the filtered load of sodium, so thiazides are less effective than loop diuretics for the treatment of heart failure. Thiazides are also weak inhibitors of carbonic anhydrase that is abundant in the proximal tubule. However, this does not contribute importantly to their natriuretic action because sodium exiting the proximal tubule is reabsorbed downstream by the loop of Henle and more distal nephron segments.

Calcium reabsorption is increased by thiazides by a direct action at the distal tubule. This may relate to enhanced activity of the Na-Ca exchanger in the distal tubule in response to decreased sodium entry. This direct tubular effect, together with volume depletion, can cause significant hypercalcemia, although it is rarely clinically significant unless primary hyperparathyroidism coexists.

Clinically significant hyponatremia can occur during treatment with thiazide diuretics. They impair the formation of maximally dilute urine through their action at the distal tubule in the renal cortex. However, unlike loop diuretics, maximum urinary concentrating ability is intact because thiazides do not interfere with the countercurrent multiplication mechanism through which the loop of Henle maintains medullary hypertonicity. Hyponatremia occurs when nonosmotic stimulation of AVP release leads to increased water reabsorption by the cortical and medullary collecting ducts.

■ **Potassium-Sparing Diuretics**

This class of diuretics includes:
- Spironolactone
- Amiloride
- Triamterene

They cause natriuresis by inhibiting sodium reabsorption through the sodium channel on principal cells in the cortical collecting tubule. This decreases the electronegativity of the tubule lumen, thereby attenuating the driving force for potassium secretion. Consequently, hypokalemia and metabolic alkalosis are avoided because potassium and hydrogen ion secretion is prevented. Patients with impaired glomerular filtration must be monitored for significant hyperkalemia and metabolic acidosis.

The efficacy of these diuretics is limited because the cortical collecting duct reabsorbs only about 2% of the filtered load of sodium. However, in combination with loop diuretics, they prevent the flow dependent increase in sodium reabsorption by the collecting tubule. This can lead to:

- Significant volume depletion
- Hypotension
- Prerenal azotemia

Spironolactone

Aldosterone stimulates sodium uptake through apical channels located on principal cells in the cortical collecting tubule. This hormone binds to a cytoplasmic receptor and the aldosterone-receptor complex is translocated to the nucleus. In a series of steps that are not completely defined, aldosterone increases sodium uptake by increasing the density of specific apical sodium channels. Electrogenic sodium reabsorption increases the electrochemical gradient for secretion of potassium and hydrogen ions.

Spironolactone is a competitive inhibitor of the cytoplasmic receptor for aldosterone. It inhibits aldosterone-stimulated sodium reabsorption and potassium secretion by preventing formation of the necessary genomic products. This natriuretic mechanism differs from other diuretics including those that are potassium-sparing (ie, amiloride, triamterene) because:

11

- Spironolactone does not bind directly to the cell membrane ion transporter
- Aldosterone enters the cytoplasm from the abluminal surface and therefore is not dependent upon glomerular filtration and tubular secretion to reach the target cell
- Spironolactone is ineffective when aldosterone levels are not elevated

The natriuretic effect of spironolactone does not reach its maximum for several days. This has been attributed to characteristics of canrenone, the major active metabolite of spironolactone. Canrenone has a two-phase elimination, with an initial half-life of 10 hours and a longer half-life of 10 to 35 hours. Excretion occurs in the urine and bile.

Patients with decompensated congestive heart failure are often unable to establish neutral sodium balance. One marker of this is a [Na]:[K] ratio less than unity in a spot urine sample. The antimineralocorticoid effects of spironolactone will cause natriuresis and reduce potassium excretion and, when titrated to an effective dose, the urinary [Na]:[K] ratio will often exceed unity.

Hyperkalemia and metabolic acidosis may occur during spironolactone therapy in patients with advanced renal insufficiency. This can be exacerbated in situations associated with impaired internal disposition of potassium (such as insulin-dependent diabetes mellitus) or during concomitant therapy with β-adrenoceptor antagonists.

Adverse symptoms of spironolactone, especially at high doses, include:
- Gynecomastia
- Menstrual irregularities
- Impotence

Some of these effects may relate to cross-reactivity of spironolactone with the testosterone and other steroid receptors.

Amiloride and Triamterene

These potassium-sparing (ie, potassium-retaining) agents do not interfere directly with endogenous aldosterone action, but directly block sodium reabsorption by the distal nephron segments thereby promoting renal K^+ and H^+ retention. These agents are often less effective than aldosterone antagonists in both their natriuretic and antihypertensive actions and are thus less useful in treating both heart failure and hypertension. They can be used cautiously in patients intolerant to aldosterone antagonists.

Diuretic Resistance and Refractory Edema

(Table 11.3)

Diuretic resistance is defined as an inadequate decrease in edema despite the administration of full doses of diuretics. When a patient fails to respond appropriately, several possibilities should be considered. It is essential to establish that the peripheral edema is related to heart failure and not caused by venous or lymphatic obstruction. Similarly, bronchospasm caused by primary bronchopulmonary disease or pulmonary embolus can mimic acute pulmonary edema.

Diuretic responsiveness can be attenuated when there is inadequate delivery of drug to the target site in the nephron. Thiazide diuretics are ineffective when renal function is moderately impaired (serum creatinine > 2 to 4 mg%); loop diuretics do not work well when the GFR is less than 5 to 10 mL/minute. In severe heart failure, gastrointestinal absorption of diuretics can be delayed and, together with impaired renal

11

TABLE 11.3 — PATHOGENESIS AND TREATMENT OF DIURETIC RESISTANCE AND REFRACTORY EDEMA

Problem	Treatment
Excess sodium intake	Measure urine sodium excretion; if > 100 meq/day then more restriction
Increased distal reabsorption	Multiple daily doses if partial diuretic response; add spironolactone or thiazide-type diuretic
Decreased diuretic entry into tubular lumen	Increase to maximum dose of loop diuretic; add spironolactone; if GFR low, then dialysis
Decreased or delayed absorption by gut	IV loop diuretic

Adapted from: Rose BD: Clinical Physiology of Acid-base and Electrolyte Disorders, 3rd edition, 1989;404. Reprinted with permission from McGraw-Hill.

function, can decrease delivery of the diuretic to the nephron and impair its action. Furosemide is highly bound to albumin and, therefore, its volume of distribution increases significantly; its bioavailability can decrease in hypoalbuminemic patients. Combined infusions of albumin and furosemide can promote natriuresis in this setting. However, this is not recommended in heart failure because the transient increase in intravascular colloid osmotic pressure can increase cardiac preload and cause acute decompensation of cardiac function and pulmonary edema.

Renal production of prostaglandins, stimulated by the high levels of angiotensin II and AVP in heart failure, attenuates tubular sodium and water reabsorption. NSAIDs inhibit prostaglandin synthesis and can blunt the response to diuretics.

As discussed above, the braking response to thiazide and loop diuretics, whereby net neutral sodium balance is maintained because natriuresis is offset by compensatory reabsorption of sodium, may be overcome by restricting dietary sodium intake and administering the diuretic twice daily. Addition of a potassium-sparing diuretic, preferably spironolactone, to a loop diuretic can overcome this braking phenomenon by enhancing the sodium load to the terminal nephron segments and by decreasing aldosterone-stimulated sodium reabsorption (and potassium secretion) in the collecting tubule. Adding a thiazide-type diuretic to a loop diuretic for this purpose is not advisable because of the marked depletion in potassium and magnesium that occurs.

Poor compliance to the diuretic or dietary regimens may be difficult to detect but, nevertheless, are also important causes of an unsatisfactory response to diuretic therapy.

Combined Therapy with ACE Inhibitor and Spironolactone

Secondary hyperaldosteronism in advanced heart failure is significant because it signals intense neurohumoral activation and identifies patients with the poorest prognosis who are most likely to benefit from treatment with ACE inhibitors (see above). Although combined therapy with loop diuretics and ACE inhibitors significantly improves symptoms, hemodynamic parameters and survival in severe heart failure, this benefit is not enjoyed by all who receive this regimen. This limited responsiveness may be due to incomplete

11

inhibition of aldosterone secretion and persistent min-eralocorticoid effects on electrolyte balance (sodium retention, potassium depletion) during ACE inhibi-tion. Support for this hypothesis was provided by a relatively small-scale study of patients with Class III-IV heart failure who had increased natriuresis and improved functional class when spironolactone was added to loop diuretics and ACE inhibitors. In addi-tion, more than 50% of the patients in the CONSEN-SUS-I Trial were treated with spironolactone and enalapril, with generally favorable outcomes.

Spironolactone therapy may also be advantageous if it decreases the extent of fibrosis that occurs during ventricular remodeling in heart failure, as has been reported in animal models of mineralocorticoid and angiotensin-mediated hypertension.

Combination therapy which includes an ACE inhibitor and spironolactone is generally avoided, however, because of concern for the increased risk of hyperkalemia and acute renal insufficiency. In the CONSENSUS-I Trial, there was no increased mortal-ity related to hyperkalemia or renal insufficiency in the enalapril-treated patients who were also taking spironolactone. However, hyperkalemia and azotemia were more commonly observed in that group as comp-ared to placebo. The issue of whether spironolactone improves survival in patients with symptomatic heart failure who are treated with ACE inhibitors and loop diuretics requires evaluation.

Mannitol

Mannitol is a polysaccharide that is not reabsorb-ed by the renal tubules and thus creates an osmotic gradient that promotes a water diuresis. By maintain-ing high urine flow, its main role is in the treatment in early phases of oliguric acute tubular necrosis and in prophylaxis against contrast nephropathy.

The associated excretion of water in excess of sodium can lead to significant hypernatremia. Furthermore, in the presence of significant renal insufficiency, mannitol excretion is impaired. This increases extracellular fluid osmolality, but decreases the serum sodium concentration by drawing water from the intracellular space into the extracellular space. This expansion of extracellular fluid volume can lead to further decompensation of cardiac function, therefore, mannitol is not recommended for the treatment of heart failure.

Adverse Effects

(Table 11.4)

Electrolyte abnormalities occur commonly during treatment with diuretics. These usually occur within two to four weeks, by which time a new steady state level of electrolyte balance has been reached. Hypokalemia is caused by:

- Decreased potassium reabsorption at the loop of Henle
- Increased potassium secretion by principal cells of the cortical collecting tubule in response to increased sodium delivery and increased renin-angiotensin-aldosterone levels
- Increased epinephrine secretion with β_2-adrenoceptor mediated redistribution of potassium into cells
- Magnesium deficit caused by decreased magnesium reabsorption in the loop

Hypokalemia and decreased cellular magnesium levels can be a serious problem in heart failure because of the related increased risk for arrhythmias. Decreases in serum potassium can be attenuated by concomitant administration of ACE inhibitors or potassium-spar-

TABLE 11.4 — ELECTROLYTE AND ACID-BASE DISTURBANCES OF DIURETIC THERAPY

Thiazides and Loop Diuretics
- Hypokalemia
- Hyponatremia (thiazides)
- Hypomagnesemia (predominantly loop diuretics)
- Hypochloremia
- Metabolic alkalosis
- Hypercalcemia (thiazides)

Potassium-Sparing Diuretics
- Hyperkalemia
- Metabolic acidosis

ing diuretics such as the aldosterone receptor agonist, spironolactone (see below).

Metabolic alkalosis is generated by the increased urinary excretion of hydrogen ions that is stimulated by secondary hyperaldosteronism, enhanced ammoniagenesis and NH_4+ secretion by the proximal tubule, and distal tubular secretion of protons. Although this is a form of chloride responsive alkalosis, sodium chloride replacement is not feasible because it can cause further deterioration of cardiac function. By reducing the dose of loop diuretic and adding acetazolamide to increase bicarbonate excretion, the metabolic alkalosis can often be corrected.

Hyperuricemia occurs commonly in heart failure and is exacerbated by volume depletion during diuretic therapy because the proximal tubular reabsorption of urate is directly related to that of sodium. Asymptomatic hyperuricemia does not require treatment, even though plasma urate levels can reach very high levels, because acute gouty arthritis and uric acid precipitation in renal tubules do not usually occur.

Ototoxicity is an important adverse effect of loop diuretics. Sensorineural hearing loss, related to inhibition of Na-K-2Cl transport in the eighth nerve usually occurs at daily doses of furosemide exceeding 1 gram. This effect is synergistic with aminoglycoside antibiotics.

Vasodilators

Heart failure is associated with neurohumoral activation that results in increased constriction of venous and arterial beds. Vasodilator therapy is designed to reduce peripheral vascular resistance and thereby enhance cardiac performance and improve symptoms. Vasodilators can be grouped into two broad categories:

1. Inhibitors of effectors that are activated in heart failure, including the:
   - Renin-angiotensin-aldosterone system (eg, ACE inhibitors)
   - Sympathetic nervous system (eg, adrenergic receptor blockers)
2. Those that decrease vascular smooth muscle tone through direct actions on:
   - Peripheral veins (eg, nitrates)
   - Peripheral arteries (eg, hydralazine, calcium channel antagonists)
   - Combined actions at both sites

The hemodynamic response to vasodilator therapy may be predicted, in part, by its site of action (Table 11.5). For example, venodilators will have desirable effects in patients primarily with symptoms related to pulmonary congestion secondary to elevated left ventricular filling pressure. In contrast, deleterious effects of venodilatation (eg, hypotension) may occur when preload has been previously optimized by di-

11

TABLE 11.5 – SITES OF VASODILATOR ACTION

Drug	Relative Action on Arteries (A) or Veins (V)
ACE Inhibitors benazepril, captopril, enalapril, fosinopril, lisinopril, ramipril, quinapril	A > V
Direct hydralazine minoxidil nitroprusside nitroglycerin isosorbide	A>>V A>>V A = V V > A V > A
Calcium Channel Antagonists diltiazem dihydropyridine, nicardipine, nifedipine, felodipine amlodipine verapamil	A>>V A>>V A>>V A>>V
α-adrenergic Blocker prazosin, terazosin, doxazosin	A = V
Dopaminergic dopamine	A > V
Adrenergic epinephrine dobutamine	A > V A > V

Reprinted with permission. Braunwald E: Heart Disease: A Textbook of Cardiovascular Medicine, 3rd edition. Philadelphia: WB Saunders, 1988.

uretic therapy, sodium restriction or in primary diastolic dysfunction in which cardiac output is extremely preload-dependent.

In the failing heart, arteriolar dilators provide afterload reduction, thereby augmenting myocardial shortening and improving systolic function. Therefore, reduction in systemic resistance, when filling pressure is elevated, is offset by a marked increased in cardiac output, and little or no decline in blood pressure. The improved baroreceptor sensitivity accounts for the decrease in heart rate commonly observed during successful treatment. The combination of venodilator and arteriolar vasodilator may also be useful when signs and symptoms of reduced perfusion and pulmonary congestion are present. By contrast, in the normal heart, cardiac output does not improve during afterload reduction and this leads to:

- Orthostatic hypotension
- Baroreceptor activation
- Reflex tachycardia

VASODILATORS THAT DECREASE NEUROENDOCRINE ACTIVITY

(In this section, the relative merits of various vasodilators will be reviewed and practical aspects of their use will be outlined.)

Angiotensin Converting Enzyme Inhibitors

11

(Table 11.6)

Results from several controlled clinical trials indicate that long-term treatment of symptomatic heart failure with angiotensin converting enzyme (ACE) inhibitors improves clinical symptoms and decreases morbidity and mortality. These favorable effects exceed those observed with other types of treatment.

TABLE 11-6 – ANGIOTENSIN CONVERTING ENZYME INHIBITORS

Drug (Trade) Name	Formulation (mg)	Total Daily Dose (mg) for Heart Failure	Pharmacokinetics		Clearance
			Peak Action/ B.P. reduction	Duration of Action	
captopril (Capoten)	12.5, 25, 50, 100	12.5-100 tid	1 hour	8 hours	renal
enalapril* (Vasotec)	2.5, 5, 10, 20	2.5 to 20 qd-bid	3 to 4 hours	12 to 24 hours	renal
lisinopril (Zestril, Prinivil)	5, 10, 20	5-20 qd	7 hours	12 to 24 hours	renal
quinapril* (Accupril)	10, 20, 40	5-20 bid	2-4 hours	12 to 24 hours	renal
ramipril* (Altace)	1.25, 2.5, 5, 10	2.5-20 qd†	2-4 hours	12 to 24 hours	renal
fosinopril* (Monopril)	10, 20	10-40 qd†	2 hours	24 hours	renal/hepatic
benazepril* (Lotensin)	5, 10, 20, 40	10 to 40 qd-bid†	2 to 6 hours	12 to 24 hours	renal/hepatic

* De-esterified in the liver to active form.
† Has no FDA approved indication for treatment of heart failure and heart failure dosages have not yet been established.

This adaptation is reproduced by permission from ASH Hypertension Handbook by Thomas G. Pickering, M.D., D.Phil., produced by the American Society of Hypertension, 1993. Publisher: LeJacq Communications, Inc., Greenwich, CT.

Furthermore, benefits of ACE inhibitor therapy have been demonstrated in asymptomatic patients with marked systolic dysfunction, including patients in whom treatment was begun shortly after myocardial infarction.

Clinical Trials of ACE Inhibitors in Symptomatic Heart Failure

Of the large clinical trials that assessed efficacy of ACE inhibitors in symptomatic patients with heart failure, five have shown significant improvement in survival.

■ CONSENSUS-I

In the Cooperative North Scandinavian Enalapril Study (CONSENSUS-I), addition of enalapril to diuretics, digoxin and non-ACE inhibitor vasodilators in patients with NYHA functional Class IV heart failure decreased total mortality (Figure 11.3). This reduction was accounted for by a 56% decrease in deaths due to progressive heart failure. However, there was no decline in the incidence of sudden death. Of the surviving patients, clinical improvement as determined by change in functional class was more common in the enalapril group than in the placebo group.

■ SOLVD (Treatment Trial)

The Studies of Left Ventricular Dysfunction (SOLVD) Treatment Trial assessed clinical outcome in patients with symptomatic heart failure treated with either enalapril or placebo in combination with digoxin, diuretics and other vasodilators. Ninety percent of patients were NYHA Class II or III, in contrast to the more severe heart failure in CONSENSUS-I. Total mortality was reduced by 16% in the enalapril group and, as in CONSENSUS-I, this primarily reflected the decrease in deaths due to progressive heart failure. In

157

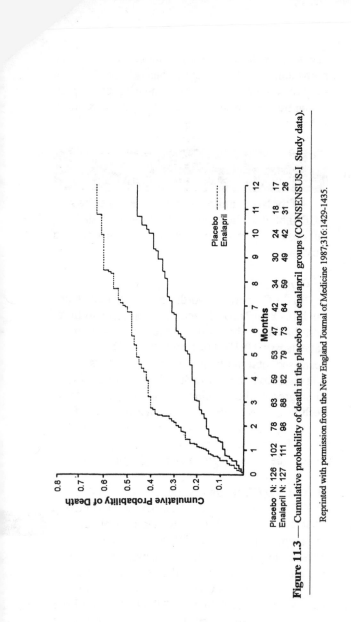

Figure 11.3 — Cumulative probability of death in the placebo and enalapril groups (CONSENSUS-I Study data).

Reprinted with permission from the New England Journal of Medicine 1987;316:1429-1435.

addition, there were fewer hospitalizations related to worsening heart failure in the enalapril group. The incidence of sudden death was not reduced by enalapril. The reductions in mortality and hospitalizations observed in this study may have been an underestimate because, during the three-year period of the study, 25% of patients in the placebo group received ACE inhibitors because of clinical deterioration.

■ V-HeFT-II

In the second Vasodilator-Heart Failure Trial (V-HeFT-II), the effects of enalapril were compared with the combination of hydralazine and isosorbide dinitrate in patients predominantly with NYHA functional Class II and III heart failure and who were taking digoxin and diuretics. There was no placebo group included in this study. Total mortality was lower in the enalapril group after two years, but did not remain significantly lower at the end of the study (Figure 11.4). In contrast to CONSENSUS-I and the SOLVD Treatment Trial, the improvement in survival was due to the reduction in sudden cardiac death rather than progressive heart failure.

By comparing these outcomes to those of the placebo control in V-HeFT-I, it is apparent that the decrease in sudden death was due to a beneficial effect of enalapril rather than a deleterious effect of hydralazine-nitrates. However, the hydralazine-nitrate group has greater improvements in ejection fraction and exercise tolerance, indicating that there is little relation between improvements in these physiologic parameters and morbidity and mortality.

■ Hy-C Trial

In this study, 117 patients with severe symptomatic heart failure, who were being evaluated for cardiac transplantation, were randomized to receive either captopril or hydralazine and nitrates. The baseline

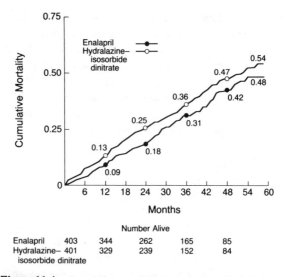

Figure 11.4—Cumulative mortality in the enalapril and hydralazine-isosorbide dinitrate treatment arms over the entire follow-up period. Cumulative mortality rates are shown after each 12-month period. For the comparison of the treatment arms after two years and overall, p = 0.016 and p + 0.08, respectively. The number of patients alive after each year is shown below the graph.

Reprinted with permission from the New England Journal of Medicine 1991;325:305.

clinical characteristics of each treatment group, including etiology of heart failure, NYHA class, and prevalence of arrhythmias and antiarrhythmic therapy, were similar. Nitrates were added to the captopril regimen during the study so that comparable numbers of patients in both groups were on nitrates during the trial.

Hemodynamic improvements were comparable in both groups. However, after 7 ± 8 months follow-up, the actuarial one year survival was higher in the captopril group (81%) than in the hydralazine group (51%). This significant improvement in survival was due to the lower rate of sudden death. For overall survival, the benefit of captopril was seen in patients

160

with serum sodium < 135 mEq/L, but not for those with sodium > 135 mEq/L. In contrast, for prevention of sudden death, captopril was beneficial in both hyponatremic and normonatremic patients. Furthermore, this reduction in sudden death rate was observed regardless of whether nonsustained ventricular tachycardia was present on Holter ambulatory electrocardiographic monitoring (Figures 11.5 and 11.6).

■ **Captopril-Multicenter Research Group**
    In this study, 92 patients with symptomatic heart failure that was refractory to digitalis and diuretics were randomized to receive either captopril or placebo. Approximately 95% of patients in each group were characterized as NYHA Class II or III. During the 90 day double-blind portion of this study, the mortality rate was significantly higher in the placebo group (21 vs. 4%) (Figure 11.7). A divergence in the survival curves became apparent after approximately 42 days of treatment. The incidence of sudden cardiac death was significantly higher in the placebo group, although the criteria for sudden death were not determined prospectively.

Clinical Trials of ACE Inhibitors in Asymptomatic Left Ventricular Dysfunction

■ **SOLVD (Prevention Trial)**
    In this arm of the SOLVD trial, patients with ejection fraction 35% or less, but without symptoms of congestive heart failure, were treated with either placebo or enalapril. Compared with placebo, fewer patients in the enalapril group developed symptomatic heart failure or required hospitalization for progressive pump failure. There was a trend toward a decrease in total mortality, primarily due to decreased cardiovascular death, although neither of these were statisti-

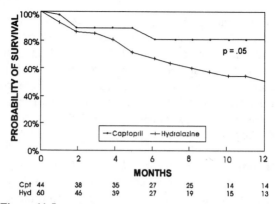

Figure 11.5 — Kaplan-Meier survival curves for the 104 patients discharged on the oral vasodilator regimen of captopril (Cpt) (n = 44) or hydralazine (Hyd) (n=60) plus isosorbide dinitrate.

Reprinted with permission. Fonarow GC, Stevenson LW, et al: Effect of direct vasodilation with hydralazine versus angiotensin-converting enzyme inhibition with captopril on mortality in advanced heart failure: the Hy-C Trial. J Am Coll Cardiol 1992;19:841-847.

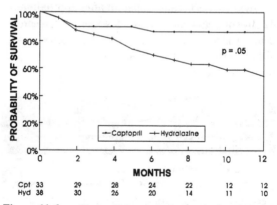

Figure 11.6 — Kaplan-Meier survival curves in the subgroup of 71 patients who remained on the initial randomized vasodilator regimen of captopril (Cpt) (n = 33) or hydralazine (Hyd) (n = 38) plus isosorbide dinitrate. Survival differences are similar to those in the larger heterogeneous group shown in Figure 11.5.

Reprinted with permission. Fonarow GC, Stevenson LW, et al: Effect of direct vasodilation with hydralazine versus angiotensin-converting enzyme inhibition with captopril on mortality in advanced heart failure: the Hy-C Trial. J Am Coll Cardiol 1992;19:841-847.

162

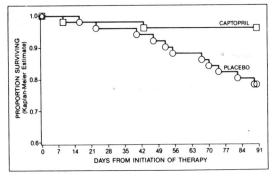

Figure 11.7 — Patient survival as a function of time.

Reprinted with permission. Newman TJ, et al: Effects of captopril on survival in patients with heart failure. Am J Med 1988;84(suppl 3A):142.

cally significant. However, the difference in mortality between placebo and enalapril groups may have been underestimated because approximately 50% of the placebo group who subsequently developed symptomatic heart failure were treated with an ACE inhibitor. When the data from the SOLVD Treatment and Prevention Trials were pooled, there were significant reductions in myocardial infarction, unstable angina and cardiac deaths in the enalapril treated patients. However, in view of the different clinical characteristics of patients in the prevention and treatment trials, this pooled analysis should be interpreted cautiously.

It is important to note that, in this trial and in the SAVE trial, survival curves did not begin to diverge for 10 to 18 months after treatment with the ACE inhibitor was begun. This suggests that, compared with the beneficial effects of ACE inhibition in symptomatic patients, the impact on mortality is delayed in asymptomatic patients because of the decrease in progressive ventricular dysfunction.

Clinical Trials of ACE Inhibitors After Acute Myocardial Infarction

■ SAVE

In the Survival and Ventricular Enlargement (SAVE) Trial, 2,231 patients with ejection fraction > 40% were randomized to treatment with either captopril or placebo within 3 to 16 days after myocardial infarction. Included in this population were patients who were asymptomatic or mildly symptomatic. The initial dose, 6.25 mg or 12.5 mg tid, was titrated upward to the maintenance dose of 50 mg tid after two weeks. The average length of follow-up was 3.5 years and approximately 80% of patients were on therapy at the target dose at the end of the study.

Compared with placebo, the captopril group had a significant reduction in total mortality, including from cardiovascular causes, and lower rates of recurrent myocardial infarction and development or progression of symptomatic heart failure requiring hospitalization (Figure 11.8). These benefits were independent of age, sex, baseline blood pressure, ejection fraction, prior myocardial infarction, or the use of other agents (thrombolytic therapy, aspirin, β-adrenergic blocker). These results demonstrate that adding captopril to standard post-MI therapies leads to additional improvements in survival and in clinical outcome in selected surivors of myocardial infarction.

■ CONSENSUS-II

In this study, patients were randomized to receive placebo or enalapril within 24 hours of a myocardial infarction and were followed for six months. Unlike the trials outlined above, ventricular performance was not assessed prior to randomization and patients were excluded if there were clear indications for ACE inhibitor therapy. There was no difference in survival

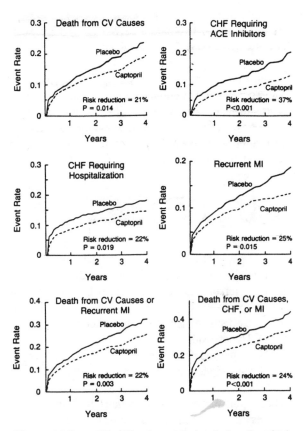

Figure 11.8 — Life tables for cumulative fatal and nonfatal cardiovascular events. CV denotes cardiovascular, CHF congestive heart failure, and MI myocardial infarction. The bottom right panel shows the following events: death from cardiovascular causes, severe heart failure requiring angiotensin-converting enzyme inhibitors or hospitalization, or recurrent myocardial infarction. For all the combined analyses, only the time to the first event was used.

Reprinted with permission from the New England Journal of Medicine 1992;327:676.

between these groups. However, there was a trend toward *increased* mortality rate due to heart failure in the enalapril group. Specifically, there was an association between hypotension, following the first dose of enalapril, and mortality. The study was stopped because of these safety concerns and because it was apparent that enalapril was unlikely to be superior to placebo with regard to six-month mortality, the primary end-point of the trial. This may have related to the higher incidence of hypotension with enalapril (25%) compared with placebo (10%).

Adverse Effects of ACE Inhibition

When cardiac output is impaired, blood pressure and glomerular filtration rate are preserved by angiotensin II mediated arteriolar vasoconstriction (see above). Interruption of these responses by ACE inhibition can cause the following common clinically significant adverse effects related to this type therapy:

- Hypotension
- Renal insufficiency
- Hyperkalemia

The extent of these complications in heart failure relates to the magnitude of activation of the renin system and to the duration of action of the ACE inhibitor. Factors that determine the activity of the renin system include the level of cardiac dysfunction and the type and dosage of concurrent diuretic therapy. Signs of neurohumoral activation, such as hyponatremia, hypokalemia, prerenal azotemia and elevated plasma renin activity in a patient with heart failure, increase the likelihood of an adverse hemodynamic response to treatment with high doses of an ACE inhibitor.

In patients with severe heart failure, ACE inhibitors with long durations of action (ie, enalapril, lisinopril) are more likely to cause prolonged episodes of hypotension. This has been associated with symptoms such as lightheadedness and syncope, and can also promote myocardial and cerebrovascular ischemia. Renal hypoperfusion, together with decreased angiotensin-mediated efferent arteriolar resistance that can occur during ACE inhibition, may lead to deterioration in GFR and decreased sodium excretion. Hyperkalemia can occur because the filtered load of potassium is reduced together with the GFR. In addition, aldosterone secretion decreases and, thus, potassium secretion is impaired. These adverse effects may be attenuated by using ACE inhibitors which have a shorter duration of action and by starting with the lowest dose. This is particularly important in patients with renal insufficiency because the primary route of excretion is the kidney.

Other adverse effects of ACE inhibitors, although not clearly related to their direct effects on angiotensin II formation, include:

- Non-productive cough
- Rash
- Dysgeusia
- Neutropenia
- Angioedema

Of these, cough is the most common, perhaps affecting up to 10 to 15% of patients. Its prevalence is uncertain but is likely underestimated. Angioedema is extremely rare, with an incidence less than 0.1%, but its onset dictates immediate discontinuation of the drug and may require additional medical attention. These effects, especially angioedema, can occur in all members of this drug class and can be expected to recur when switching to a different ACE inhibitor.

ACE Inhibitors

The use of ACE inhibitors in heart failure will:
- Improve cardiac performance by:
  - Increasing cardiac output
  - Reducing ventricular end-diastolic pressure
  - Reducing systemic vascular resistance
- Improve survival
- Improve New York Heart Association functional class:
  - Less dyspnea and fatigue
  - Increased exercise capacity
- Conserve potassium and magnesium
- Correct hyponatremia (when combined with furosemide)
- Reduce ventricular arrhythmias
- Reduce emergency interventions and hospitalizations
- Reduce myocardial oxygen requirements in coronary disease

Adrenoceptor Antagonists

■ **β-adrenoceptor Antagonists** (Table 11.7)

Heart failure is characterized by:
- Excess activation of the sympathetic nervous system
- Decreased number and affinity of myocardial β-adrenoceptors
- Impaired contractile response to β-adrenergic agonists

Results from several studies suggest that chronic β-adrenoceptor blockade may improve hemodynamic function and clinical outcome in patients with heart failure, particularly in those with idiopathic cardiomyopathy and ischemic heart disease. Treatment with β-adrenoceptor blockers increased:

- β-adrenergic receptor density
- The contractile response to a β-agonist infusion
- Ejection fraction

However, improvements in systolic function also occurred without associated upregulation of β_1-adrenoceptors. Therefore, other mechanisms may contribute to the clinical improvement reported in some patients with heart failure during treatment with antagonists. For example, renin secretion is suppressed during β-blockage and so this, or attenuation of other neurohumoral mechanisms activated in heart failure, might account for its beneficial effects.

Despite the reports of favorable clinical responses to β- adrenoceptor blockade, there is a significant risk for clinical deterioration related to worsening heart failure. This is most likely due to the negative inotropic effects of these drugs. These adverse effects may be ameliorated with the use of newer agents currently being evaluated.

α-adrenoceptor Antagonists

(Table 11.8)

Treatment with α-adrenoceptor antagonists improves the hemodynamic profile in heart failure. For example, prazosin produces a balanced effect on arterioles and venous capacitance with associated decreases in peripheral vascular resistance and blood pressure. As a consequence, stroke volume and cardiac output increase, and exercise tolerance improves. However, attenuation of these hemodynamic effects has been reported during long-term treatment with α-adrenoceptor antagonists. This may be related to

11

TABLE 11.7 — β-ADRENERIC ANTAGONISTS

Drug (Trade) Name	Formulation (mg)	Daily Dose (mg)	Mode of Action			Pharmacokinetics			
			β₁	β₂	ISA	Peak Action	Duration of Action	Clearance	

Drug (Trade) Name	Formulation (mg)	Daily Dose (mg)	β_1	β_2	ISA	Peak Action	Duration of Action	Clearance
Cardioselective								
metoprolol (Lopressor, Toprol XL)	50, 100 50, 100, 200	50 to 200 bid 50 to 200 qd	++ ++	+ +	0 0	1 hour 6 hours	8 to 12 hours 24 hours	hepatic hepatic
atenolol (Tenormin)	50, 100	50 to 100 qd	++	+	0	2 to 4 hours	12 to 24 hours	renal
betaxolol (Kerlone)	10, 20	10 to 40 qd	++	+	0	3 hours	24 to 36 hours	hepatic/renal
Nonselective								
propranolol (Inderal, Inderal LA)	10, 20, 40, 60, 80, 60, 120, 160	20 to 120 bid 120 to 340 qd	+++ +++	++ ++	0 0	1 hour 6 hours	6 to 12 hours 12 to 24 hours	hepatic hepatic
timolol (Blocadren)	5, 10, 20	10 to 20 bid	++	++	0	1 to 2 hours	6 to 12 hours	hepatic

nadolol (Corgard)	20, 40, 80, 120, 160	40 to 320 qd	++	++	0	2 to 4 hours	24 hours	renal
penbutolol (Levatol)	20	20 to 40	++	++	0	2 hours	12 to 24 hours	hepatic
ISA								
pindolol (Visken)	5, 10	5 to 30 bid	++	++	++	1 hour	6 to 12 hours	hepatic/renal
carteolol (Cartrol)	2.5, 5	2.5 to 10 qd	++	++	++	2 hours	12 to 24 hours	hepatic/renal
acebutolol (Sectral)	200, 400	200 to 400 bid	++	±	+	2 hours	12 to 18 hours	hepatic/renal
Combined α_1, β labetalol (Normodyne, Trandate)	100, 200, 300	100 to 400 bid	++	++	0	2 hours	8 to 12 hours	hepatic

Reproduced by permission from ASH Hypertension Handbook by Thomas G. Pickering, M.D., D.Phil., produced by the American Society of Hypertension, 1993. Publisher: LeJacq Communications, Inc., Greenwich, CT.

11

TABLE 11.8 — α-ADRENERGIC ANTAGONISTS

Drug (Trade) Name	Formulation (mg)	Daily Dose (mg)	Mode of Action α_1	Mode of Action α_2	Peak Action	Duration of Action	Clearance
Nonselective phenoxybenzamine (Dibenzyline)	10	10 to 40 bid, tid	++	++	6 hours	36 hours	urine
Selective prazosin (Minipress)	1, 2, 5	1 to 5 tid, qid	+	0	2 hours	6 hours	hepatic
terazosin (Hytrin)	1, 2, 5, 10	1 to 20 qd	+	0	2 hours	24 hours	hepatic
doxazosin (Cardura)	1, 2, 4, 8	2 to 16 qd	+	0	3 hours	24 hours	hepatic

Pharmacokinetics spans the columns Peak Action, Duration of Action, and Clearance.

Reproduced by permission from ASH Hypertension Handbook by Thomas G. Pickering, M.D., D.Phil., produced by the American Society of Hypertension, 1993. Publisher: LeJacq Communications, Inc., Greenwich, CT.

increased norepinephrine levels or sodium retention that occur during treatment with these agents. It may also be related to the short half-life of prazosin since more sustained benefit might occur with doxazosin or terazosin.

Furthermore, in the V-HeFT-I trial in which long-term survival of patients treated with either prazosin or combination hydralazine-nitrates were compared with placebo, improvement in survival was found in the hydralazine-nitrate group but not in the prazosin group. Therefore, α-adrenoceptor antagonists do not have a primary role in the chronic treatment of heart failure.

Direct Vasodilators

- **Nitrovasodilators** (Table 11.9)
  Potent vasodilators include:
  - Nitroprusside
  - Nitroglycerin
  - Isosorbide dinitrate

They relax vascular smooth muscle by stimulating production of cGMP, which is formed when their active metabolite (nitric oxide) stimulates guanylate cyclase (Figure 11.9). The intermediary metabolism of nitrovasodilators to nitric oxide is not completely understood, however, they must enter vascular smooth muscle in order to produce nitric oxide. This mechanism of nitric oxide mediated vasodilatation is the same as that which is utilized by endogenous vasodilators (ie, acetylcholine, bradykinin). However, the mechanism of nitric formation differs from that of endothelium-dependent vasodilating substances, in which nitric oxide is produced in endothelial cells by the conversion of arginine to citrulline, and then diffuses across the endothelium into the vascular smooth muscle cell.

11

TABLE 11.9 – DIRECT VASODILATORS

Drug (Trade) Name	Formulation	Daily Dose	Pharmacokinetics			
			Peak Action	Duration of Action	Clearance	
nitroglycerin **Transdermal Delivery** (Nitro-Dur, Transderm Nitro, Nitrodisc, Minitran, Deponit NTG)	0.1 to 0.6 mg/hour	0.2 to 0.8 mg/hour	> 2 hours	10 to 12 hours	hepatic/RBC	
Intravenous (Nitro-Bid, Tridil, Nitrostart)	5 to 100 mg/ampoule	5 to 640 Kg/min	< 3 to 5 min	< 10 min	hepatic/RBC	
Ointment (Nitro-Bid)	2% ointment	7.5 to 45 mg q6 to q8 hours	< 3 to 5 min	4 to 6 hours	hepatic	

174

Nitrolingual Spray	0.4/metered dose	< 2 to 3/15 min	1 to 4 min	30 to 60 min	hepatic
Tablets					
(Nitro-Stat)	0.15, 0.3, 0.4, 0.6 mg	< 2 to 3/15 min	1 to 4 min	30 to 60 min	hepatic
(Nitrong)	2.6, 6.5 mg	2.6 to 26 mg tid	10 min	4 to 6 hours	hepatic
Other Vasodilators:					
hydralazine (Apresoline)	10, 25, 50, 100 mg	10 to 100 mg tid-qid	1 hour	6 hours	hepatic
minoxidil (Loniten)	2.5, 10 mg	2.5 to 20 mg bid	2 hours	12 hours	hepatic
nitroprusside (Nipride)	50 mg/5 mL vial	0.3 to 10 µg/kg/min	1 to 2 min	10 min	hepatic/renal

Reference: Physicians' Desk Reference, 47th edition. Montvale, NJ: Medical Economics Data, 1993.

11

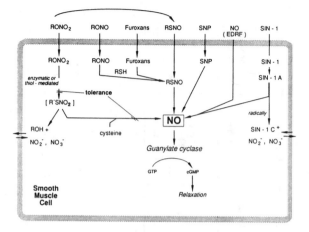

Figure 11.9 — Proposed scheme of soluble guanylate cyclase activation with respect to the different pathways of NO formation from nitrovasodilators. Abbreviations: EDRF, endothelium-derived relaxing factor; Furoxans, 3.4 disubstituted furazan-2-oxides; NO, nitric oxide; RONO, organic nitrate; RSH, thiol; RSNO, nitrosothiol; SIN-1, active metabolite of molsidomine; SNP, sodium nitroprusside.

Reprinted with permission. Lewis BS, Kimchi A: Heart Failure Mechanisms and Management. New York: Springer-Verlag,1991;251.

Tolerance to the vasodilating effects can occur during continuous use. This relates to the decreased availability of free sulfhydryl groups and, consequently, decreased formation of nitrosothiol intermediates that are required for nitric oxide synthesis from organic nitrates. Tolerance to nitrovasodilators can be avoided by adjusting the daily dosing schedule so that nitrates are withheld for eight to twelve consecutive hours each day. Nitroprusside does not utilize these nitrosothiol metabolites for nitric oxide formation and this may account for the lack of cross-tolerance with other nitrovasodilators.

Nitroprusside: This is a balanced vasodilator which reduces tone in arterioles and veins. It is administered intravenously and has a short duration of action. It can be particularly useful in the treatment of decompensated heart failure in the setting of mitral and aortic regurgitation, and following cardiac surgery. Hypotension, related to its vasodilator action, should be avoided by careful titration, but is reversible within 10 minutes after discontinuing the infusion.

Another adverse effect is excess accumulation of thiocyanate, a metabolite of nitroprusside, which can occur within a few days of continuous infusion. Thiocyanate is excreted by the kidney and therefore patients with renal insufficiency are at higher risk for thiocyanate toxicity, manifested by:

- Convulsion
- Psychosis
- Abdominal pain
- Muscle twitching
- Dizziness
- Hypothyroidism

Serum thiocyanate levels should be measured in patients at increased risk and maintained below 6 mg%.

Nitroglycerin: This vasodilator acts predominantly on the venous and pulmonary arterial beds, with less effect on the resistance vessels unless high doses are used. It is available in several formulations, including:

- Sublingual
- Topical
- Intravenous

It decreases preload and myocardial oxygen consumption when pulmonary capillary pressure is high. However, it may cause hypotension and reduce cardiac output in heart failure when left ventricular filling pressure is low. Intravenous nitroglycerin also has an important role in the setting of acute myocardial infarction, where it has been shown to decrease mortality and reduce infarct expansion.

Isosorbide dinitrate: This is a long-acting nitrate that can be taken sublingually or orally. Its potential adverse effects are similar to those described for nitroglycerin.

In the V-HeFT-I Trial, survival was improved in patients with heart failure treated with a combination of isosorbide dinitrate (40 mg qid) and hydralazine (75 mg qid). In addition, exercise tolerance and heart failure symptoms were improved by this treatment. However, in a subsequent study (V-HeFT-II), enalapril improved survival more than hydralazine-isosorbide, suggesting that ACE inhibitors may be preferred therapy (see above).

■ **Hydralazine**

This vasodilator acts primarily on the arteriolar smooth muscle. Favorable hemodynamic responses are more likely to occur in heart failure with greater degrees of left ventricular enlargement and peripheral vascular resistance. In the V-HeFT trials, prognosis was directly related to the treatment-related increase in ejection fraction that occurred in combination with isosorbide dinitrate.

Its onset of action after an oral dose is approximately 20 to 30 minutes. Side effects include:
- Flushing
- Headaches
- Fluid retention

A lupus-like syndrome has been described in approximately 15% of patients at daily doses of 400 mg, with a higher percentage having titers for antinuclear antibodies. This phenomenon is more common in the slow acetylator phenotype, who metabolize hydralazine at a decreased rate. This lupus-like syndrome resolves after discontinuation of hydralazine. The intravenous preparation is no longer available.

■ Minoxidil

Minoxidil is predominantly an arteriolar vasodilator. It is not frequently utilized in the treatment of heart failure because it commonly causes fluid retention which requires increasing doses of diuretics. In addition, hypertrichosis is an adverse effect that occurs commonly and is undesirable for many patients.

■ Calcium Channel Antagonists (Table 11.10)

In general, all vasodilators have favorable short-term effects on cardiac performance and symptoms. However, the direct vasodilators, particularly the calcium channel antagonists, are often not well tolerated and they do not improve survival in advanced heart failure. To the contrary, early use of calcium channel antagonists after myocardial ischemia or infarction has been associated with increased mortality rates. These adverse effects may relate to the increases in plasma renin activity and plasma catecholamines that occur during direct vasodilator therapy. In addition, calcium channel antagonists have negative inotropic effects that can further impair ventricular performance. These adverse effects may be less pronounced with some of the newer agents, although additional studies will be required.

Common side effects include:
- Palpitation
- Flushing
- Edema
- Constipation
- Gingival hyperplasia

11

■ Verapamil

Verapamil has the strongest negative inotropic effect of all the calcium blockers that are currently in

TABLE 11.10 — CALCIUM CHANNEL ANTAGONISTS

| Drug (Trade) Name | Formulation (mg) | Daily Dose (mg) | Pharmacokinetics | | | Tissue Selectivity | | |
			Peak Action	Duration of Action	Clearance	Vasodilation	Myocardial Depression	A-V Node
Dihydropyridine nifedipine (Procardia, Adalat) (Procardia XL)	10, 20 30, 60, 90	10 to 20 qid 30 to 90 qd	1/2 hour 6 hours	4 to 6 hours 24 hours	hepatic hepatic	++ ++	+ +	0 0
nicardipine (Cardene) (Cardene SR)	20, 30 30, 45, 60	20 to 40 tid 30 to 60 bid	1 to 2 hours 1 to 4 hours	6 to 8 hours 8 to 12 hours	hepatic hepatic	++ ++	0 0	0 0
isradipine (Dynacirc)	2.5, 5	2.5 to 5 bid	1 to 2 hours	8 to 12 hours	hepatic	++	0	0
felodipine (Plendil)	5, 10	5 to 20 qd	3 to 5 hours	24 hours	hepatic	++	+	+

	2.5, 5, 10	2.5 to 10	6 to 12 hours	24 hours	hepatic	++	0	0
amlodipine (Norvasc)	2.5, 5, 10	2.5 to 10	6 to 12 hours	24 hours	hepatic	++	0	0
Miscellaneous								
verapamil								
(Isoptin, Calan)	40, 80, 120	80 to 120 tid	1 to 2 hours	6 to 8 hours	hepatic	+	+++	+++
(Isoptin SR, Calan SR)	180, 240	180 to 240 qd-bid	7 to 8 hours	20 to 24 hours	hepatic	+	+++	+++
(Verelan)	120, 180, 240	120 to 240 qd	7 to 9 hours	20 to 24 hours	hepatic	+	+++	+++
diltiazem								
(Cardizem)	30, 60, 90, 120	30 to 120 tid	2 to 3 hours	6 to 8 hours	hepatic	+	+	+
(Cardizem SR)	60, 90, 120	60 to 120 bid	6 to 11 hours	12 to 18 hours	hepatic	+	+	+
(Cardizem CD)	180, 240, 300	180 to 300 qd	10 to 14 hours	20 to 24 hours	hepatic	+	+	+
(Dilacor XR)	180, 240	180 to 480 qd	4 to 6 hours	24 hours	hepatic	+	+	+

Reference: Physicians' Desk Reference, 48th edition. Montvale, NJ: Medical Economics Data, 1994.

11

use. Hemodynamic deterioration and exacerbation of heart failure symptoms has been reported in patients with elevated pulmonary capillary pressure. Therefore, the afterload reduction with verapamil appears to be insufficient to offset its negative inotropic effect and so it should be avoided in patients with heart failure.

■ **Nifedipine**

In contrast to verapamil, nifedipine is a potent vasodilator which acutely decreases systemic vascular resistance and may improve cardiac performance. However, 20 to 30% of patients with NYHA functional Class IV heart failure will have worsening symptoms after a single dose. Long-term use in heart failure has been associated with increased cardiac filling pressure, heart rate and body weight. This clinical deterioration has been associated with reflex neurohumoral activation (increased renin and catecholamine secretion) that occurs during treatment. These adverse effects of nifedipine may be ameliorated by concurrent administration of β-adrenoceptor antagonists and, therefore, are not related to its negative inotropic effects. Furthermore, nifedipine has not been shown to have beneficial effects on survival and, therefore, should not be used as primary therapy for heart failure.

■ **Diltiazem**

Diltiazem may have a lesser negative inotropic effect than either nifedipine or verapamil. However, its use in heart failure has been associated with clinical deterioration which may relate to decreases in heart rate observed during treatment. In light of these findings, diltiazem should not be used as primary treatment for heart failure.

Positive Inotropic Agents

■ **Digitalis** (Table 11.11)

Chronic digitalis therapy has been shown to have beneficial effects in patients with advanced heart failure due to systolic dysfunction. In the intact heart, digitalis improves contractility, shifting the ventricular function curve so that at any given level of ventricular filling pressure, more stroke work is generated. In the failing heart, this leads to reduced oxygen consumption because of the related decreases in end-diastolic volume and wall stress. In the nonfailing heart, there is little or no increase in cardiac output despite increased myocardial contractility. This reflects changes in other determinants of cardiac performance, including increased peripheral vascular resistance (afterload). Patients who benefit most from digoxin tend to have:

- More chronic and severe heart failure
- Dilated left ventricle
- Reduced ejection fraction
- S_3-gallop

Although digitalis compounds have been used for two centuries, their mechanisms of action are not entirely understood. By inhibiting Na-K$^+$-ATPase digoxin:

- Increases cytosolic sodium and calcium
- Enhances:
  - Myocardial contractility
  - Stroke volume
  - Exercise capacity

11

Digoxin also decreases conduction velocity through the atrioventricular node, and thereby can provide additional benefits by slowing the ventricular response rate in patients with atrial fibrillation and atrial flutter.

TABLE 11.11 – CARDIAC GLYCOSIDE PREPARATIONS

Agent	Gastrointestinal Absorption	Onset of Action	Peak Effect	Average Half-Life	Principal Metabolic Route (Excretory Pathway)	Average Digitalizing Dose		Usual Daily Oral Maintenance Dose*
						Oral	Intravenous	
Digoxin	55 to 75%	15 to 30	1½ to 5 hours	36 to 48 hours	Renal; some gastro-intestinal excretion	1.25 to 1.50 mg	0.75 to 1.00 mg	0.125 to 0.25 mg
Digitoxin	90 to 100%	25 to 120	4 to 12 hours	7 to 9 days	Hepatic; renal excre-tion of metabolites	0.70 to 1.20 mg	1.00 mg to 1.2 mg	0.05 to 0.3 mg

*Maintenance dose is determined by clinical indications and digoxin level.

Reference: Physicians' Desk Reference, 48th edition. Montvale, NJ: Medical Economics Data, 1994.

In addition to its direct augmentation of cardiac contractility, digoxin also has other salutary effects on neurohormonal responses in heart failure (Figure 11.10). It decreases renin secretion, possibly by directly increasing cytosolic calcium in juxtaglomerular cells, which leads to a fall in angiotensin II and aldosterone levels. Digoxin also improves baroreceptor sensitivity, and consequently reduces sympathetic outflow. Therefore, therapeutic benefits of digitalis in heart failure include its impact on neurohumoral mechanisms as well as its direct effects on the myocardium.

Digoxin, either alone or in combination with diuretics and ACE inhibitors, can be highly effective in treating congestive heart failure. Withdrawal of digoxin from patients treated with combination therapy, including ACE inhibitors, results in:

- Decreased exercise tolerance
- Worsening NYHA functional classification
- Decreased ejection fraction
- Increased heart rate
- Lower quality-of-life score

This indicates that the beneficial effects of digoxin are not supplanted ACE inhibitors and that there is a therapeutic advantage of combination therapy which includes each of these drugs.

Pharmacokinetics: The most commonly used digitalis preparation is digoxin. The pharmacokinetic properties of digoxin and digitoxin are outlined in Table 11.11. Gastrointestinal absorption of digoxin is incomplete when given after meals or when given with nonabsorbable antacids. The steady-state, total body content of a therapeutic dose of digoxin for an adult is approximately 10 µg/kg. This correlates to a serum concentration of approximately 1.5 ng/mL. Assuming 75% absorption of a tablet, the oral loading dose is approximately 1 mg for a 70 kg individual administer-

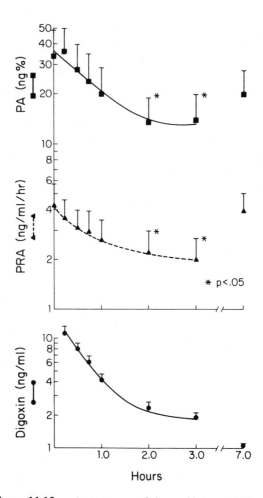

Figure 11.10 — Acute response of plasma aldosterone (PA) and plasma renin activity (PRA) to bolus administration of digoxin (0.50 mg) in patients not receiving oral digoxin therapy. The serum digoxin concentration is also given. *p < 0.05 vs. baseline.

Reprinted with permission from The American Journal of Cardiology 1992;69:144G.

ed over a 24 hour period. Parenteral loading and maintenance doses are approximately 75% of the oral doses. Digoxin is excreted primarily by the kidney and its half-life increases from approximately 36 hours to 4.4 days in patient's renal failure.

Distribution of digoxin is affected by several factors. Importantly, it is not bound by adipose tissue and so doses should be calculated according to lean body mass. Fifty percent of digitalis is bound to Na-K-ATPase receptors in skeletal smooth muscle and physical activity can significantly decrease the serum concentration. In addition, several medications that are used to treat heart failure interfere with the distribution and excretion of digoxin.

The uses of the serum digoxin measurement are outlined in Table 11.12. A major error in the use of this level is the failure to wait for equilibration, which requires 12 hours following an oral dose. For this reason, it is useful to have the patient take the digoxin dose in the evening prior to the morning blood sampling. Patients who have had suboptimal subjective and objective responses to digoxin with steady-state serum levels < 1 ng/mL can improve significantly when the level is increased to 1.5 ng/mL.

Digitalis toxicity: The incidence of digitalis toxicity has reportedly decreased with the availability of serum measurements. However, the prevalence is increased in certain circumstances outlined in Table 11.13.

There are no specific arrhythmias that are diagnostic of digitalis toxicity. However, toxicity should be suspected in patients with atrial fibrillation in whom A-V junctional tachycardia occurs and is recognized clinically as paradoxical regularization of the ventricular rate. Supraventricular tachycardia that originates from A-V nodal reentry (ie, PAT with block) and A-V junctional block with Wenckebach periodicity

TABLE 11.12 — INDICATIONS FOR SERUM RADIOIMMUNOASSAY OF DIGOXIN

- Validate dose
- Assess:
  - Compliance
  - Bioavailability
  - Effect of renal function on excretion
  - Effects of other drugs on elimination
  - Effects of hemodynamic changes
  - Failure to respond
- Prevent toxicity
- Diagnose toxicity

Reprinted with permission from The American Journal of Cardiology 1992;69:104G.

TABLE 11.13 — FACTORS ASSOCIATED WITH INCREASED RISK FOR DIGITALIS TOXICITY

- Renal insufficiency
- Electrolyte abnormalities:
  - Hypokalemia
  - Hypomagnesemia
  - Hypercalcemia
- Hypothyroidism
- Advanced pulmonary disease
- Pharmacokinetic interactions with other drugs, eg:
  - Quinidine
  - Verapamil
  - Amiodarone
- Pharmacodynamic interactions with other drugs (eg, sympathomimetic agents)

Reprinted with permission from The American Journal of Cardiology 1992;69:110G.

may also be evidence of digoxin toxicity. Electrolyte disturbances increase the risk of digitalis toxicity; hypokalemia and hypercalcemia can exacerbate digitalis induced arrhythmias. Hyperkalemia may occur after a massive digitalis overdose because the inhibition of Na-K-ATPase leads to the translocation of potassium from the intracellular to extracellular space.

Extracardiac manifestations of toxicity are nonspecific but are common in affected patients. Symptoms include:
- Anorexia
- Fatigue
- Nausea
- Vomiting

A visual disturbance of halos around bright objects is a less common, but somewhat more specific symptom.

The key to successful treatment of digitalis toxicity is early recognition that an arrhythmia may be related. Treatment should include cautious administration of potassium, especially if serum levels are low or even in the normal range. Digoxin-specific F(ab) fragments of high affinity, polyclonal antibodies remove digitalis rapidly from myocardial and other tissue binding sites. They have a high volume of distribution and their effect is effectively irreversible. The response rate is rapid, with a mean initial response 19 minutes after F(ab) fragment infusion. Failure to respond is most commonly attributed to ineffective dosing or moribund clinical state before F(ab) administration.

Other pharmacologic interventions are less effective than F(ab) fragment therapy. Phenytoin and lidocaine can be effective treatment. Direct current countershock may be hazardous and is not advisable. Steroid binding resins (ie, cholestyramine, colestipol) interrupt the enterohepatic circulation of digitoxin by trapping it in the intestine, but the effect is insufficient

11

in the case of life-threatening toxicity. Hemodialysis is ineffective because of the high degree of protein binding and volume of distribution. Ventricular pacing with an endocardial catheter electrode is usually effective, although ventricular standstill not responsive to pacing has been reported.

Non-Digitalis Inotropic Agents

The use of positive inotropic agents other than digitalis is largely limited to the hospital intensive care unit and the more severe forms of congestive heart failure. Many of these agents are still experimental, showing ambiguous survival data and a formidable array of side effects, and are not yet approved by the FDA for chronic oral therapy. Table 11.14 lists the more commonly used non-digitalis inotropic agents.

■ Sympathomimetic Amines

Dopamine (Table 11.15)

Dopamine is the endogenous biosynthetic precursor of norepinephrine. It stimulates cardiac β_1-adrenoceptors directly and this effect is blocked by β_1-adrenoceptors antagonists. In contrast dopamine-mediated vasodilatation in the renal, coronary, cerebral and mesenteric beds is mediated by a specific DA_1-receptor that increases cAMP activity in postjunctional vascular smooth muscle. Dopamine stimulation of prejunctional DA_2-receptors contributes to its vasodilating action by inhibiting release of norepinephrine from sympathetic nerves.

The effects of dopamine on vascular resistance and arterial pressure are dose-dependent (Figure 11.11). At low doses (< 2 µg/kg/min), selective vasodilatation of renal, coronary and mesenteric beds occurs. At intermediate doses (2 to 5 µg/kg/min), myocardial contractility and cardiac output increases accompa-

TABLE 11.14 — ADRENERGIC RECEPTOR ACTIVITY OF SYMPATHOMIMETIC AMINES

Agonist	α	β₁	β₂
Norepinephrine	++++	++++	0
Epinephrine	++++	++++	++
Dopamine*	++++	++++	++
Isoproterenol	0	++++	++++
Dobutamine	+	++++	+
Phenylephrine	++++	0	0
Methoxamine	++++	0	0

*Causes renal and mesenteric vasodilatation by stimulating dopaminergic receptors.

Reproduced with permission from the New England Journal of Medicine 1979;300:18.

nied by either a decrease or no change in heart rate. At higher doses (5 to 10 g/kg/min), peripheral vascular resistance increases because of vasoconstriction mediated by α_1-adrenoceptors and serotonergic receptors.

Dobutamine

Dobutamine is a positive inotropic drug that stimulates both β- and α-adrenoceptors, but has predominantly β_1- and α_1- adrenergic activity. In heart failure, these actions tend to increase myocardial contraction, stroke volume and cardiac output while reducing systemic vascular resistance so that blood pressure remains relatively constant. Dobutamine causes redistribution of cardiac output to coronary and skeletal muscle beds. It has been reported to have favorable

11

TABLE 11.15 — Non-Digitalis Positive Inotropic Agents

Agent	Mechanism	Comment
Norepinephrine (intravenous only)	β_1-, α_1-agonist	Increases cyclic AMP and stroke force but also has α_1-stimulation for intense vasoconstriction. Not appropriate for severe heart failure, but useful in cardiogenic shock for restoring blood pressure
Epinephrine (intravenous only)	β_1-, β_2- and α_1-agonist	As above, but may cause tachycardia and arrhythmia. Not recommended for congestive heart failure but useful in managing cardiac arrest
Isoproterenol (intravenous only)	β_1-, β_2-agonist	β_1 inotropy combined with β_2 vasodilatation. However, tendency for tachycardia and arrhythmia may reduce rather than increase cardiac output. Initial bolus: 0.02 to 0.06 mg; initial infusion: 5 µg/min

Dopamine (intravenous only)	DA_1-, DA_2-, β_1-, α_1-, α_2-agonist. Epinephrine precursor	In low doses (< 2 μg/kg/min) improves blood flow and natriuresis. In high doses (> 2 μg/kg/min) increases contractility with peripheral vasoconstriction and venoconstriction
Dobutamine (intravenous only) (Dobutrex)	β_1-, β_2- and α_1-agonist	Increases stroke volume and peripheral vasodilatation. Slight venoconstriction. Lengthy infusions (> 72 hours) induce tolerance. Dose 2.5 to 15 μg/kg/min
Amrinone (intravenous only)	Phosphodiesterase-III inhibition	Increases stroke volume plus vasodilation to reduce preload. Can replace dobutamine in the event of intolerance. Loading dose: 0.75 mg/kg; maintenance infusion: 5 to 10 μg/kg/min

Reference: Physicians' Desk Reference, 48th edition. Montvale, NJ: Medical Economics Data, 1994.

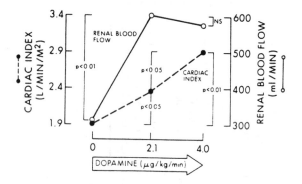

Figure 11.11 — Changes in cardiac index and renal blood flow in response to ascending doses of dopamine.

hemodynamic effects in patients with acute myocardial infarction and heart failure without increasing the extent of infarction or provoking further ischemia. Dobutamine is not a selective renal vasodilator, but can be used together with low-dose dopamine to augment renal blood flow in heart failure.

Phosphodiesterase Inhibitors

Unlike the sympathomimetic amines, which exert their inotropic effect by increasing formation of cAMP through β-adrenoceptor stimulated adenylate cyclase activity, phosphodiesterase inhibitors increase intracellular cAMP levels by decreasing its breakdown to AMP. Development of these compounds for clinical use has been disappointing because of the increased incidence of morbidity and mortality associated with their use in clinical trials.

At the present time, amrinone is the only approved phosphodiesterase inhibitor. It is only available for intravenous use, and at low doses (10 μg/kg/min) is an effective afterload reducing agent. It should be avoided in patients with low blood pressure or in whom peripheral vascular resistance is not increased.

Vesnarinone is an orally active agent that was shown to decrease morbidity and mortality in patients with heart failure after administration for six months. This drug has several actions, including inhibition of phosphodiesterase, increased ion channel activity with increases in intracellular sodium and increasing intracellular calcium. However, it has a low toxic:therapeutic dose ratio, with an increased mortality rate observed at a dose only twice that at which beneficial effects were observed.

Anticoagulation

Systemic and pulmonary thromboembolic events occur relatively commonly in patients with congestive cardiomyopathy, with an incidence in 10 to 20% reported in several clinical studies. In some of those studies, this risk increased even further in patients with atrial fibrillation and markedly impaired systolic function.

These observations have led to the use of prophylactic anticoagulation in patients with heart failure. However, in the V-HeFT trials thromboembolism was relatively uncommon and its incidence was not decreased by anticoagulation with warfarin. In that study, this risk was not increased by atrial fibrillation or other factors that have been associated with thromboembolic events in patients without heart failure.

These discordant findings, together with the 10% risk of clinically significant bleeding related to warfarin, heighten the controversy regarding the role of anticoagulants or antiplatelet agents in the prophylaxis and treatment of thromboembolic events in heart failure. A long-term prospective trial of the efficacy

and safety of anticoagulant therapy in patients with
heart failure is required to provide clearer indications
for its use. Until then, cautious use of anticoagulants
should be considered in patients with severe heart
failure unless there is a contraindication to their use.

Antiarrhythmic Therapy

Sudden death is common in patients with heart
failure. The incidence of sudden death has been
related to ventricular tachycardia. However, mortality
rates increased during treatment with Type I antiarrhythmic agents during a prospective evaluation,
possibly reflecting their proarrhythmic or negative
inotropic effects (Table 11.15).

There are data to suggest that decreasing neurohumoral activation may reduce the risk of sudden
death in patients with congestive cardiomyopathy
(Table 11.16). In V-HeFT-II, enalapril treatment was
associated with fewer episodes of ventricular
tachycardia and sudden death than combination
hydralazine-nitrates therapy. Captopril therapy decreased the incidence of sudden death when compared
with placebo (Captopril Multicenter Research Group)
and hydralazine (Hy-C Trial). However, several other
large placebo-controlled clinical trials of ACE inhibitor therapy have not found a decrease in sudden death,
even though mortality from other cardiovascular etiologies declined significantly. ∂-adrenoceptor blockers
decrease sudden death in the setting of myocardial
infarction and may also have benefit in dilated
cardiomyopathy, although the mechanism responsible
for this effect is not established.

Taken together, the data are insufficient to support the use of specific antiarrhythmic agents for the
routine treatment of patients with heart failure in
whom asymptomatic, nonsustained ventricular
tachycardia is detected. In some patients, additional

TABLE 11.16 — STUDIES OF ARRHYTHMIC DEATH IN HEART FAILURE

Trial	Drug	Total Death	Arrhythmic Death
CONSENSUS-I	enalapril	decrease	no change
V-HeFT-I	prazosin, hydralazine-nitrates	decrease	N/A
V-HeFT-II	enalapril, hydralazine-nitrates	decrease	decrease
SOLVD therapy	enalapril	decrease	no change
SOLVD prevention	enalapril	±	no change
Hy-C	captopril	decrease	decrease
Captopril Multicenter Group	captopril	decrease	decrease
CAST-I	encainide, flecainide	increase	increase
CAST-II acute chronic	moricizine	increase no change	increase no change

Modified from: Greene HL: Arrhythmias in congestive heart failure. Clinical Cardiology 1992;15(suppl I):I-13–I-21. This table was reprinted with permission of Clinical Cardiology Publishing Co., Inc.; Box 832; Mahwah, NJ 97430-0832 USA.

attempts should be made to optimize treatment of the underlying cardiomyopathy, including adequate diuresis, afterload reduction and correction of electrolyte and acid-base disturbances. Patients with symptomatic ventricular arrhythmias should be considered for further evaluation and treatment with a specific antiarrhythmic regimen.

CARDIAC TRANSPLANTATION

Cardiac transplantation is the most effective form of therapy for terminal heart failure, with 85% survival after one year. In addition, approximately 80% of patients improve to NYHA functional Class I or II. This is in comparison to a first year mortality rate of 40% in patients with NYHA Class IV who are treated with ACE inhibitors. More than 3,000 heart transplants were performed worldwide in 1990, with its use limited by the availability of organ donors.

The primary indication for heart transplantation is progressive heart failure in a younger patient who has not responded to medical therapy. The most common etiologies include coronary artery disease and idiopathic cardiomyopathy.

Following transplantation, patients are prone to recurrent heart failure. The most common causes include:
- Early right ventricular overload and tricuspid regurgitation
- Acute rejection
- Restrictive disease and related diastolic dysfunction
- Allograft coronary artery disease

The latter is considered to be immunogenic and long-term studies suggest that it occurs in as many as 50% of patients five years after transplantation. It may not be associated with angina because the heart is denervated. The specific treatment of heart failure in the transplant patient will depend upon the specific etiology.

REFERENCES

1. Cohn J: Current therapy of the failing heart. Circulation 1988;78:1099-1107.

2. Smith TW, Braunwald E, Kelly RA: Management of heart failure. In: Heart Disease: A Textbook of Cardiovascular Medicine. Braunwald E (ed). Philadelphia: WB Saunders, 1988;chapter 17.

3. Rose BD: Clinical use of diuretics. In: Clinical Physiology of Acid-base and Electrolyte Disorders, 3rd edition. Rose BD (ed). New York: McGraw-Hill, 1989;chapter 17.

4. Rose BD: Regulation of the effective circulating volume. In: Clinical Physiology of Acid-base and Electrolyte Disorders, 3rd edition. Rose BD (ed). New York: McGraw-Hill, 1989;chapter 17.

5. Pecker M: Pathophysiologic effects and strategies for long-term diuretic treatment of hypertension. In: Hypertension: Pathophysiology, Diagnosis and Management. Laragh JH, Brenner BM (eds). New York: Raven Press, 1990;chapter 137.

6. Wilcox CS: Diuretics. In: The Kidney, 4th edition. Brenner BM, Rector FC (eds). Philadelphia: WB Saunders, 1991;chapter 45.

7. Shackelton CR, Wong NLM, Sutton RAL: Distal (potassium-sparing) diuretics. In: Diuretics: Physiology, Pharmacology and Clinical Use. Dirks JH, Sutton RAL (eds). Philadelphia: WB Saunders, 1986;chapter 6.

8. van Vliet AA, et al: Spironolactone in congestive heart failure refractory to high-dose loop diuretic and low-dose angiotensin converting enzyme inhibitor. Am J Cardiol 1993;71:21A-29A.

9. Dahlstrom U, Karlsson E: Captopril and spironolactone therapy in patients with refractory congestive heart failure. Curr Ther Res 1992;51:235-248.

11

10. Weber KT, Brilla CG: Pathologic hypertrophy and cardiac interstitium: fibrosis and renin-angiotensin-aldosterone system. Circulation 1991;83:1849-1865.

11. Chattergee K: Vasodilator therapy for heart failure. In: Drug Treatment of Heart Failure. Cohn JN (ed). New York: Yorke Medical Books, 1983;chapter VII.

12. Packer M: Pathophysiology of heart failure. Lancet 1992; 340:88-92.

13. Yusuf S, Garg R: Design, results and interpretation of randomized, controlled trials in congestive heart failure and left ventricular dysfunction. Circulation 1993;87(suppl VII):VII-115–VII-121.

14. The CONSENSUS-I Trial Study Group: Effects of enalapril on mortality in severe congestive heart failure. N Engl J Med 1987;316:1429-1435.

15. SOLVD Investigators: Effects of enalapril on survival in patients with reduced left ventricular ejection fraction and congestive heart failure. N Engl J Med 1991;295:293-302.

16. Captopril Multicenter Research Group: A placebo-controlled trial of captopril in refractory chronic congestive heart failure. J Am Coll Cardiol 1983;2:755-763.

17. Newman TJ, Maskin CS, Dennick LG, et al: Effects of captopril on survival in patients with heart failure. Am J Med 1988;64(suppl 3A):140-144.

18. Fonarow GC, Chelimsky-Fallick C, Stevenson LW, et al: Effect of direct vasodilatation with hydralazine versus angiotensin converting enzyme inhibition with captopril on mortality in advanced heart failure: The Hy-C Trial. J Am Coll Cardiol 1992;19:842-850.

19. Pfeffer MA, et al: Effect of captopril on mortality and morbidity in patients with left ventricular dysfunction after myocardial infarction. N Engl J Med 1992;327:669-677.

20. The CONSENSUS-II Trial Study Group: Effects of the early administration of enalapril on mortality in patients with acute myocardial infarction. N Engl J Med 1992;327:678-684.

21. Furburg CD, Campbell RWF, Pitt B: (Letter to the editor) N Engl J Med 1993;328:967.

22. SOLVD Investigators: Effect of enalapril on mortality and the development of heart failure in asymptomatic patients with reduced left ventricular ejection fraction. N Engl J Med 1992;327:685-691.

23. Yusuf S, et al: Effect of enalapril on myocardial infarction and unstable angina in patients with low ejection fractions. Lancet 1992;340:1173-1178.

24. Cohn JN, et al: Effect of vasodilator therapy on mortality in chronic congestive heart failure: results of a Veterans Administration cooperative study (V-HeFT). N Engl J Med 1986; 314:1547-1552.

25. Cohn JN, et al: A comparison of enalapril with hydralazine-isosorbide dinitrate in the treatment of chronic congestive heart failure. N Engl J Med 1991;325:303-310.

26. Packer M, et al: Comparison of captopril and enalapril in patients with severe chronic heart failure. N Engl J Med 1986;315:847-853.

27. Fowler M: Controlled trials with beta-blockers in heart failure: metoprolol as prototype. Am J Cardiol 1993; 71:45C-53C.

28. Feelisch M, Noack E: The in-vitro metabolism of nitro-vasodilators and their conversion into vasoactive species. In: Heart Failure: Mechanisms and Management. Lewis BS (ed). Berlin: Springer-Verlag, 1991;241-255.

29. Packer M: Pathophysiological mechanisms underlying the adverse effects of calcium channel-blocking drugs in heart failure. Circulation 1989;80(suppl IV):IV-59–IV-67.

30. Kimchi A, Lewis BS: Calcium channel antagonists in the management of heart failure. In: Heart Failure: Mechanisms and Management. Lewis BS (ed). Berlin: Springer-Verlag, 1991;241-255.

31. Packer M, et al: Withdrawal of digoxin from patients with chronic heart failure treated with angiotensin converting enzyme inhibitors. N Engl J Med 1993;320:1-7.

11

32. Lewis RP: Clinical use of serum digoxin concentrations. Am J Cardiol 1992;69:97G-107G.

33. Kelly RA, Smith TW: Recognition and management of digitalis toxicity. Am J Cardiol 1992;69:108G-119G.

34. Leier CV: Current status of non-digitalis positive inotropic drugs. Am J Cardiol 1992;69:120G-129G.

35. Feldman AM, et al: Effects of vesnarinone on morbidity and mortality in patients with heart failure. N Engl J Med 1993;329:149-155.

36. Mudge GH: Strategies to manage the heart failure patient after transplantation. Clin Cardiol 1992;15(suppl I):I-37–I-41.

37. Fuster V, et al: The natural history of idiopathic dilated cardiomyopathy. Am J Cardiol 1981;47:525-531.

38. The Cardiac Arrhythmia Suppression Trial (CAST) Investigators: Effect of encainide and flecainide on mortality in a randomized trial of arrhythmia suppression after myocardial infarction. N Engl J Med 1989;321:406-412.

39. Dunkman BW, et al: Incidence of thromboembolic events in congestive heart failure. Circulation 1992;87(suppl VI):VI-94–VI-101.

12   Putting It All Together: Treatment of CHF

(see Section #11, Pharmacologic Therapy,
for a more detailed discussion)

AFTERLOAD REDUCTION

Angiotensin Converting Enzyme Inhibitors

Over the past 20 years, important new insights have emerged for understanding the pathophysiology of congestive heart failure which have resulted in meaningful therapeutic advances.   Central to this understanding has been the elucidation of the strategic role of the renin-angiotensin-aldosterone axis in the neurohumoral response to impaired cardiac output (Figure 12.1). As outlined previously in this mono- graph (see Sections #5 and #6 regarding *Sodium and Volume Homeostasis*), the renin system is activated to maintain arterial pressure and flow. This compensa- tion becomes maladaptive because angiotensin-in- duced systemic vasoconstriction augments afterload and further embarrasses the failing heart. Chronically elevated angiotensin and aldosterone:

- Induce sodium-volume expansion
- Increase preload
- Add to the cardiac burden

12

The importance of the renin system in the patho- physiology of congestive heart failure is highlighted by the significant reductions in mortality and cardio- vascular morbidity reported in several large clinical

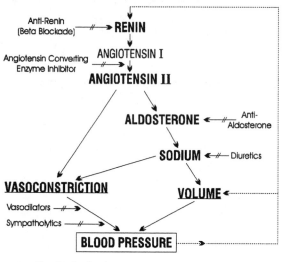

Figure 12.1 — Vasoconstriction-volume hypothesis and the renin axis.

trials in which affected patients were treated with angiotensin converting enzyme (ACE) inhibitors. This points to the measurement of plasma renin activity (PRA) as a useful marker for predicting whether an individual patient will have a beneficial response to an ACE inhibitor – this is analogous to the important role of plasma renin profiling in hypertension as a useful method for selecting the right antihypertensive medication. Indeed, a number of clinical trials have shown that ACE inhibitors are less effective in CHF patients in whom the renin system has not been activated (ie, PRA < 2.0 ng/mL/hr). However, there has not yet been a large prospective clinical trial designed to assess the effects of ACE inhibitors on mortality in patients with CHF and low plasma renin activity.

Accordingly, an important clinical question is when to begin treatment with ACE inhibitors. Evidence is accumulating which suggests that asymptomatic patients with reduced ejection fraction (EF < 40%) may benefit from ACE inhibitor therapy, particularly in the period shortly after a myocardial infarction (see Section #11, *Pharmacologic Therapy*). This therapy can prevent cardiac remodeling while reducing cardiac work, all direct consequences of afterload reduction and natriuresis caused by reduction of angiotensin and aldosterone levels. Moreover, unlike diuretic therapy, potassium and magnesium balance is maintained and exercise capacity is less impaired, thereby contributing to a better quality of life.

ACE inhibitor therapy with captopril has a special place in treating the patient with dyspnea because symptomatic relief and clinical efficacy can be rapidly established. Peak blood levels are achieved within an hour of an oral dose of captopril (12.5 to 25 mg) and this can be associated with dramatic relief of dyspnea and pulmonary congestion. The patient may then continue with captopril or switch to a longer acting ACE inhibitor if there is no significant decline in renal function or hypotension.

In the asymptomatic patient, additional pharmacologic therapy (ie, diuretics, digitalis, nitrates) may not be required. However, these latter medications become important for the management of symptomatic heart failure.

The risk of acute renal failure with ACE inhibitors is increased in patients who are treated concomitantly with diuretic, particularly if they have evidence for markedly decreased effective circulating volume, including prerenal azotemia, hyponatremia and hypotension prior to starting the ACE inhibitor. Concurrent use of other nephrotoxic drugs increases further the risk of acute renal failure. Most notable are nonsteroidal anti-inflammatory agents (NSAIDS) which through their inhibition of prostaglandins, promote both acute renal failure and severe hyperkalemia. Therefore, to reduce the risk of acute renal failure and hyperkalemia prior to administering the first dose of an ACE inhibitor:

- Reduce the diuretic dose for 24 to 48 hours
- Discontinue all nephrotoxic drugs (ie, NSAIDs)
- Begin with low doses of short-acting ACE inhibitors: captopril 6.25 to 12.5 mg bid or tid for one week; titrate to maintenance dose of 25 to 50 mg bid or tid
- Follow serum electrolytes, creatinine, BUN weekly during initial one to two weeks
- If no hypotension or decline in renal function, may switch to a longer acting preparation (ie, enalapril), then reassess renal function

Aldosterone production, and the related sodium retention, is increased in CHF as a consequence of renin-angiotensin activation. Diuretics enhance aldosterone secretion by further increasing renin secretion, especially in advanced stages of CHF, and this in turn can attenuate the natriuretic response and exacerbate the signs and symptoms of CHF. This vicious cycle can be interrupted by ACE inhibitors through the related reduction in angiotensin II formation. However, the renin-angiotensin system is often dramatically elevated in CHF, and ACE inhibitors can promote an additional reactive rise in renin release by the kidney. This marked elevation in PRA (ie, 50 to 100 ng/mL/hr) can overcome the pharmacologic inhibition of angiotensin converting enzyme by these drugs (ie, captopril and enalapril). Consequently, angiotensin II is formed, afterload increases, aldosterone production is enhanced, and sodium retention occurs even though the patient is presumably on a therapeutic dose of an ACE inhibitor.

Thus, it is evident that ACE inhibitors may be ineffective in patients with CHF for at least two reasons:

- Low PRA (< 2 ng/mL/hr) prior to initiation of ACE inhibitor
- Rise in PRA during therapy overcomes ACE inhibition

Thus, an individual patient may not improve clinically while on an ACE inhibitor either because the renin system is not stimulated prior to therapy or because it is stimulated in excess of the degree of ACE inhibition. In the latter case, increasing the dose of the ACE inhibitor may complete the blockade of angiotensin II formation and lead to a more favorable clinical response.

Measurement of 24-hour urinary aldosterone provides an additional index of ACE inhibition that compliments PRA, because angiotensin II is the major stimulus for aldosterone excretion (Figure 12.2). Therefore, if both the PRA and urinary aldosterone levels are *high* while on an ACE inhibitor, ACE inhibition is incomplete and the dose should be increased. If the PRA is high but the urinary aldosterone level is low, ACE inhibition is complete despite the rise in PRA, and it is unlikely that there will be additional benefit from an increased dose.

When PRA is *low* during therapy with an ACE inhibitor, increasing the dose is unlikely to lead to clinical improvement. Instead, increasing doses of diuretics, nitrates, digitalis and positive inotropic agents (dobutamine, vesnarinone) are more likely to result in clinical improvement.

Thus, as with hypertensive patients in whom renin profiling is useful for the assessment of secondary etiologies, treatment selection and stratification of cardiovascular risk, congestive heart failure measurement of plasma renin activity can also provide a useful guide for selecting and titrating medications.

12

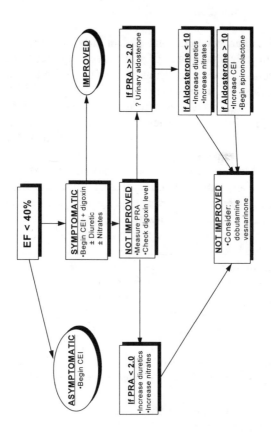

Figure 12.2 — Guide to therapy of congestive heart failure. (CEI = angiotensin converting enzyme inhibitor)

The most common side effect associated with ACE inhibitors is cough. It is characterized as nonproductive, with a "tickle" sensation that may be more common at night. It is important to distinguish this cough from that associated with pulmonary congestion, in which dyspnea is also prominent. Patient descriptions of the ACE inhibitor cough range from it being a minor annoyance to intolerable. Some find it less common at lower doses or with shorter acting preparations, although it appears to be related to the drug class rather than these other features. There is no known long-term toxicity related to the cough and it has not been related to other more serious side effects such as angioedema.

Hydralazine

Hydralazine is an arteriolar vasodilator that, when combined with a nitrovasodilator (ie, isosorbide dinitrate) effectively reduces morbidity and mortality in patients with CHF. However, it is less effective than enalapril at reducing mortality and so should be used primarily in patients in whom ACE inhibitors are not tolerated.

The effective dose range is 25 to 100 mg tid or qid. However, a lupus-like syndrome is more likely to occur at total daily doses of approximately 400 mg.

β-adrenergic Receptor Antagonists

Congestive heart failure is characterized by intense neurohumoral stimulation that, in addition to increased activity of the renin-angiotensin-aldosterone system, also includes heightened adrenergic activity. Evidence for the latter includes high levels of plasma catecholamines and impaired baroreceptor reflexes. Consequently, β_1-adrenoceptor antagonists (ie, metoprolol 25 to 50 mg bid), when used at low doses in patients with mild-to-moderately impaired function, can improve cardiac performance. However, in patients with more severe disease, the related negative inotropic effects can lead to further decompensation of CHF.

PRELOAD REDUCTION

Diuretics

Diuretics are indicated in patients with symptomatic congestive heart failure in whom dietary sodium restriction is insufficient. Loop diuretics are most effective because they inhibit sodium reabsorption by the medullary thick ascending limb, normally a major site of sodium reabsorption.

Reduction in body weight is the most sensitive index of a diuretic response. In the absence of edema, a daily weight loss of 0.5 to 1.0 kg together with objective findings (ie, rales, S_3-gallop) are useful indices of clinical response. In the presence of peripheral edema, or in acute pulmonary edema, more aggressive diuresis may be necessary.

Diuretic responsiveness can be reduced when there is inadequate delivery of diuretic to the nephron target site of action. This may occur because:
- Gut absorption is impaired
- Hypoalbuminemia increases volume of distribution
- Glomerular filtration is reduced below a critical level:
  - Loop diuretics: < 5 to 10 mL/min
  - Thiazide-type diuretics: < 25 to 30 mL/min
- Concurrent use of NSAIDs impairs formation of prostaglandins which have natriuretic and diuretic properties
- Poor compliance by the patient

The response to diuretics may also be attenuated by a "braking phenomenon" whereby net neutral sodium balance is maintained because natriuresis is offset by compensatory reabsorption of sodium. The mechanism of this response is not completely understood, but it can be overcome by restricting dietary sodium intake and by administering the diuretic dose twice daily.

Secondary hyperaldosteronism, in which aldosterone secretion is stimulated by the high renin-angiotensin levels common in advanced CHF treated with loop diuretics, has important implications for assessing cardiovascular risk and selecting treatment regimens. In CONSENSUS-I, mortality was increased in patients in the placebo group in whom aldosterone concentration exceeded the median level. Furthermore, in the enalapril group, mortality decreased *only* in patients in whom aldosterone levels were elevated above the median prior to treatment. Enalapril did not decrease mortality in those with aldosterone concentrations at or below the medial level. In subsequent studies, adding spironolactone to the regimen of patients with NYHA III-IV CHF that was refractory to therapy with combination loop diuretics and ACE inhibitors resulted in significantly increased natriuresis and improved functional class. Hyperkalemia and prerenal azotemia were rarely of significant magnitude to warrant discontinuation of spironolactone or the ACE inhibitor. Thus, spironolactone is an under appreciated, effective diuretic in which complications such as hypokalemia and hypomagnesemia are circumvented, especially in patients with CHF and secondary hyperaldosteronism. Side effects (ie, gynecomastia, menstrual irregularities) are uncommon at the low doses that are often sufficient in the treatment of CHF.

Spironolactone has a relatively slow onset of action, so that a clinical response may not be apparent for approximately two weeks and a maximal may not be observed for several weeks. An initial dose of 25 mg/d is often sufficient, but can be titrated up to 50 to 75 mg bid. Higher doses are more commonly associated with side effects and may not offer additional therapeutic benefit. Thus, spironolactone is most effective in the chronic management of CHF rather than for treating acute, severe decompensated congestive heart failure.

Nitrovasodilators

Nitroglycerin and related nitrovasodilators reduce preload primarily by dilating venous and pulmonary arterial beds. Pharmacodynamics of nitrate therapy are characterized by:
- Rapid onset of action
- Tolerance when used continuously

Nitrate intolerance, defined as an attenuated response to a previously effective dose, can be avoided by maintaining a 12 hour nitrate-free period each day (ie, during sleep).
Several preparations are available, including:
- Topical
- Oral
- Sublingual tablet and aerosol

Side effects include:
- Headache, flushing, palpitations
- Tachycardia
- Hypotension

Nitrate-induced hypotension is more likely to occur in the setting of excessive diuresis and can precipitate acute renal failure, especially during concomitant use of ACE inhibitors. This requires reduction in the dose of nitrates and other vasoactive medications. Initial doses of commonly used preparations include:

- Nitroglycerin patch: 0.2 mg/hr
- Isosorbide dinitrate: 10 mg tid

POSITIVE INOTROPIC AGENTS

Digitalis

Digoxin has recently been shown to have beneficial effects when combined with ACE inhibitors. In addition to its effects on myocardial contractility, recent studies have demonstrated that digitalis also improves baroreceptor responsiveness and inhibits renin secretion. There are no firm guidelines regarding when to initiate therapy with digitalis, although its arrays of actions suggest that it may be of benefit in mild-to-moderately symptomatic patients, especially if they are also treated with an ACE inhibitor.

The digitalis dose can be titrated according to the serum level, with the upper limit of the therapeutic level for digoxin at 1.6 ng/mL. Dose adjustments are required for patients with renal insufficiency and for a variety of concurrently used medications (see Section #11, *Pharmacologic Therapy*). Several factors increase the risk for digitalis toxicity, including hypokalemia and hypomagnesemia. These electrolyte disturbances are common during diuretic therapy and should be identified and corrected prior to beginning digitalis.

Commonly effective initial doses include a loading dose of 0.75 to 1.0 mg within 24 hours, followed by 0.125 to 0.25 mg/d. A serum digoxin level should be drawn approximately 12 hours after a maintenance dose.

12

Dobutamine

Dobutamine is a positive inotropic drug that stimulates both β- and α-adrenoceptors, which in congestive heart failure tends to improve cardiac performance and reduce peripheral vascular resistance. It is particularly useful in patients with severe, decompensated CHF who are not responsive to other therapies.

It can only be administered intravenously. The dosage range is 2.5 to 15 µg/kg/min.

Amrinone

Amrinone is a phosphodiesterase inhibitor that is parenterally administered. Its positive inotropic effects are mediated by the related increase in cAMP.

It is administered as a loading dose (0.75 µg/kg) followed by a maintenance infusion at 5 to 10 µg/kg/min.

Vesnarinone

Vesnarinone is an orally active agent that was recently shown to decrease morbidity and mortality in patients with congestive heart failure. It has several actions, including phosphodiesterase inhibition. However, it has a relatively low toxic-therapeutic threshold, such that morbidity and mortality were *reduced* after six months in those treated with 60 mg/d and *increased* in those treated with 120 mg/d. The long-term effects of vesnarinone are not known.